BECOMING
NURSEY

From Code Blues to Code Browns,
How to Care for Your Patients and Yourself

By Kati Kleber, BSN RN

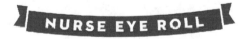

NURSE EYE ROLL

BookBaby Publishing

BookBaby.com

Disclaimer

This book is about my personal nursing experiences and does not reflect the views of any past or current employers, coworkers, patients, or their loved ones.

This book is for informational purposes only.

In all circumstances, refer to your facility's policies and procedures, as that will always be what guides your practice. The information provided in this book is meant to supplement—not replace—your existing knowledge.

Any discussion about patients is purely for learning purposes and HIPAA compliant, as identifying details have been changed to protect their privacy.

You will note that some of the material in here has come from my blog. I have taken a few old blog posts, dusted them off, and enhanced them greatly. Why not all-new material, you ask? As I was combing through some of my previous material, I realized that some of it is essential foundational information, and to leave it out would be a disservice to those beginning their nursing journey.

This book is meant to be a comprehensive guide to learn how to work and live as a nurse. I don't want people to feel that they have to search through my blog for pieces of information to see the full picture. So if you come across something that seems familiar, it may be that you have read it before its nursey makeover.

ABOUT THE AUTHOR

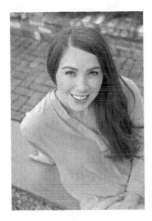

Hello there! My name is Kati and I am a bedside critical care nurse in Charlotte, North Carolina. I live with my husband, who makes me laugh until I cry every single day and is so handsome it hurts. He's my best friend. I also live with the two handsomest pups you ever did see. I couldn't ask for anything more.

I love going to farmer's markets, watching and quoting *the Office*, and spooning my dogs after a tough day. My favorite food is one I didn't make or clean up. I'm a rock star on the nursing unit, but have no idea how to buy fashionable clothes or decorate my home. I typically outsource these tasks to more skillful individuals.

I love Christ with all that I am. A Proverbs 31 Woman is who I aspire to be.

For Christ.

TABLE OF NURSEY CONTENTS

ACKNOWLEDGEMENTS

I want to take a moment to thank every single patient and their loved ones, that I've had the honor of caring for.

I want to thank every coworker and members of nursing leadership that have helped me become a better nurse with each and every shift.

I want to thank my husband for editing every single word I write and constantly encouraging me.

I want to thank my parents for putting me through nursing school, believing in me, and supporting every thing I've done.

I want to thank all of my non-nursing friends and family for having to listen to my constant nurse-talk over the years. I especially want to thank my non-nursing friends that have not only endured listening to it, but who have given me sound advice and encouragement with every single step.

I want to thank my nursing school professors and classmates for dealing with me during that trying time.

I want to thank each and every one of you that have read my blog, followed me on Twitter, and supported me throughout this crazy journey. I sincerely appreciate your support and encouragement. It means more than you know.

I want to thank God for putting in me a never-ending desire to care for patients and support fellow nurses.

Seriously guys, from the bottom of my nursey heart, thanks.

Alright, let's get nursey!

INTRODUCTION

I was clueless when I graduated from nursing school.

One would assume that after thousands of dollars, many sleepless nights, exam after exam over hundreds of pages worth of material, and one big scary board exam, I would be an awesome nurse.

I think we all assume that people who go to nursing school suddenly know how to be a good nurse when they graduate. Prospective nurses assume that; so do employers. And most importantly, so do patients.

However, this could not be further from the truth. New graduate nurses walk on the unit their first day terrified, ill-prepared, and overwhelmed.

If you had handed me an angiocath (what we use to start IV's) the first day on the job, I would have looked at you like a dog does when you give it a command it doesn't know. Head tilt, eyebrow furrow and all.

The problem is, there is a big gap between being handed a license and actually doing the work of a nurse. It is so large, 50 bariatric hospital beds stretched end-to-end could fit there.

After going to school for four years, one would assume that I would know what I was doing when I started the job for which I specifically went to school. I was terrified that I would hurt a patient out of my ignorance and felt so alone. Somehow, I convinced myself that everyone knew what they were doing except for me. All through nursing school and during my first year as a nurse, I scoured the Internet for help. And I said a few prayers.

Dear Lord, please tell me someone is going through this too? Please tell me someone is going home crying once every few weeks... please tell me someone is terrified every time they have to talk to a doctor... *please tell me someone has no clue how to delegate to these nursing assistants that have been on the unit for 10 years, and I just got here last week...*

Alas, I couldn't find much online. Yes, there are your textbooks and a few other books with many stories from the bedside, but none that were both entertaining and informative. I couldn't find anyone with whom I could identify to give me real, practical advice and guidance without fluff.

I just wanted someone that was still practicing at the bedside, that hadn't graduated too long ago, to just tell me like it is. I wanted to know what it's really like to be a nurse. I wanted to know the little details they don't tell you about in school.

Sadly enough, I could not find a book to adequately suit my needs. I trudged along anyway, hoping I'd be able to figure it out as I went.

I graduated with my bachelors of science in nursing (BSN) in 2010 from a small Midwestern nursing school. After graduation, I landed a job on a cardiovascular and thoracic surgical step-down unit and worked there for two years. I then started working in a critical care unit and have worked full time on that unit since. I truly have found my nursing niche: geriatrics, brains, and intensive care. Glory be to God.

It took one graceful preceptor—an entire unit of fantastic coworkers, a new graduate residency program, and an entire year of working at the bedside to feel confident and competent in my nursing care.

How crazy is that?

So after I got to a point where I felt like I knew what I was doing, I decided that I wanted to provide that information to those of you going through the same struggle.

In 2013, I started an anonymous nursing blog, Nurse Eye Roll. I started tweeting (@NurseEyeRoll) and blogging (nurseeyeroll.com) about just that: things you need to know to do your job effectively and efficiently, all while maintaining your sanity.

Why Nurse Eye Roll, you ask? When I was thinking of a name for my blog, this was the first name that came to mind and I just couldn't get it out of my head. If you've been a nurse for 10 minutes, you've done a "nurse eye roll."

You know, when you've spent 20 minutes meticulously changing a dressing and the doctor comes by, pulls it off to look at the wound, and leaves. Or when you have to hang three different drips, none of which are compatible, and your IV pump dies. Or when you and your trusty CNA just gave your patient the best bed bath ever and as you walk out of the room, you smell that you have to start all over again.

As nurses on the frontlines, we deal with so many crazy and ridiculous things that sometimes, all you can do is smile, shake your head, and roll your eyes.

(Now, on to the next nursey task—you're already behind!)

After posting and tweeting advice, the response from the online nursing community was more profound than I ever expected... so many people felt what I felt, this hopeless lost feeling during school, for about a year, and sporadically thereafter. After coming out with posts about dealing with school, calling doctors, time management, and encouragement, I started to receive notes, messages, and emails across all of my various social media platforms about how helpful my information was to them.

That is the purpose of this book. It's a collection of a few of my posts that I dusted off and enhanced greatly, new stories, and new advice to those of you walking through this nursey world. I hope that if it was dark and scary before, this book will be your flashlight. Hopefully this book will be the practical advice and encouragement you need to help you become the best nurses you can be.

Let's do this.

CHAPTER 1

Gandalf the Grey, BSN RN

"So, why do you want to be a nurse?"

Don't you hate that question? People ask it in nursing school interviews, job interviews, on applications, and just in general life conversation. For the first five years of my nursing journey, I didn't have a good answer to that question.

For a passionate nurse, I seemed pretty *not* passionate, huh?

My generation has grown up to believe that everyone gets to do what they desire and somehow make enough money to pay for a large beautiful HGTV-ready home, and car that costs more than my yearly salary... and that we're all entitled to it.

Alas, that is not reality. Many personally and professionally satisfying jobs do not come with a salary that accommodates such living. And if miraculously it does, typically there are years of paying down debt, which will not allow you to enjoy the fruit of your labor.

I wasn't one of those people who always knew what they wanted to do with their lives. I didn't know which path to take freshmen year of college and didn't have this burning desire in me to become something specific. I envied those who did. My friends who knew they wanted to be a teacher, a pilot, a CPA, a doctor, etc., all had a passion for it and nothing else would satisfy their professional urge.

If you are one of those people who just knew within you which career was for you, please consider that a blessing gracefully given. Please be thankful for that. The rest of us are out there, trying not to go into financial ruin, attempting to figure out what we should do with the rest of our lives.

I was very aware of the need to quickly make a decision about the path I was going to take, but painfully unaware of which path I wanted to take. With so many options, so much potential debt in front of me, and little time, I made not a passionate decision, but a *practical* decision to go with nursing.

Honestly, this was my thought process: I like teaching and I like health/medicine, so nursing makes sense, right? I won't pretend it was more complicated than that. That's all I had to go on.

I started taking prerequisites at a junior college and prayed that it was the right decision. I prayed I even could get into nursing school. I prayed that I wouldn't hate it.

Surprisingly enough, I quickly found out that I loved nursing. Learning disease processes, caring for patients, and understanding the 'why' behind everything was so intriguing to me. I couldn't get enough.

Somehow I got through nursing school. Coffee, prayer, and living in the building literally next door to all of my classes (and therefore waking up approximately eight minutes before each class) were my saving grace.

Throughout school, I discovered that while I loved nursing, I wasn't sure if it loved me. When you're taking your nursing courses, you think you know what being a nurse is going to be like, but you don't *really* know yet. I was praying that once I got through school not only would I enjoy the real world of nursing, but that I'd love it enough to stay in the field for decades to come.

When I started working at the bedside, I discovered not only did I like nursing, but it liked me back and we got along well. Even as a young and naïve nurse just surviving each shift, I was able to have a profound impact on my patients. I discovered that you don't have to be one of those expert nurses with years of experience to take good care of someone.

In order to do the job of a nurse, you have to have an awareness and knowledge of technical things (equipment, computers, medications, diagnoses and conditions, etc.) because clearly that is important to practicing safe patient care. This is what I call the "black" part of nursing.

However, there is this side of nursing that is not technical or in nursing textbooks. I call this the "white" part of nursing. That's when you can walk into a room and just feel the emotional climate. You can tell when you need to be comforting, motivating, supportive, or even silent. You are able to command respect from your patient and their loved ones while still being soft and gentle. You're able to walk into the room of a patient with a completely different cultural background and still bond greatly with them. You're able to get patients and their families to trust you quickly.

It's putting them both together that truly makes a good nurse. I call it being "grey."

It is in this grey blend of the black of nursing (technical stuff) and the white of nursing (creative/social/emotional) in which the good nurses live. They know enough technical information to be safe and efficient. They have enough social, emotional, and creative awareness to make their patients feel safely cared for, and somehow know how to get things done efficiently.

Having wisdom, grace, and discernment in terrible situations isn't something that everyone carries within them. Not everyone can explain complex medical conditions to a crying patient. Compassionate care is something we assume all nurses do— simply because they are nurses. Once you get out there, you'll realize that is not the case.

Being a grey nurse is not automatic. It takes going through some rough situations and learning from them. It means gracefully accepting constructive criticism and allowing it to make you a better nurse. It means checking your ego at the door. It means caring about the big picture. It means knowing and acknowledging the fact that while this may be just another day at work for us, it is a profound time in our patients' lives, and our needs are not the priority.

The Good Grey Nurses

I've been very blessed in my short career as a nurse to be exposed to some amazing nurses. There are some nurses that just get it. They understand that big picture. They know it's not about them; it's always about the patient, and that fact is evident in everything they do.

You know them when you see them. You're probably thinking about those nurses that work on your unit right now.

They're the ones who can take on a heavy patient load, be in charge, and are somehow on time with everything. They're the ones who know when they need to drop everything and be there for a patient during a really rough moment. They're the ones who patients request by name. They're the ones who you go to first when you have a bad feeling about one of your patients. They're the ones with whom you, and your patients, feel *safe*.

There is something about a good nurse. Having a nursing license and job doesn't make you a good nurse. Working for 30 years doesn't make you a good nurse. It's not about being a good IV starter or being best friends with all of the physicians. It's not about having a commanding presence or knowing all of the answers to the 900 questions you get asked each shift.

While all of these things are important, it's not all there is. It's so much less defined and measurable than that. It isn't measured in letters after your name, certifications, professional affiliations, or by climbing the clinical ladder. It's something you feel when you see a good nurse care for their patients. It's that security you see in their patient's eyes when they come in to care for them. It's that nurse whose patient's family member will finally go home to sleep and shower because they know their loved one is cared for with that nurse.

Good nurses breathe instinct. They breathe discernment. Good nurses can pick out seemingly insignificant things about a patient, interpret an intricate clinical picture, somehow predict a poor outcome, and bring it to the doctor's attention, literally saving someone's life.

Did you read that? Save someone's *life*. I have seen the lives of patients spared because of something that their nurse, their *good* nurse, first noticed.

And then there's that heart knowledge that good nurses have that blows me away even more.

They are those nurses who always know the right thing to say. They know how to calm an apprehensive and scared mother enough to let them take care of her son.

They know how to re-explain the worst news a husband is ever going to hear because it didn't quite make sense when the doctor said it 15 minutes ago. And they know how to comfort and reassure him when they see it click in his mind that his wife is forever gone.

They know when to just sit and listen to a man tell his entire life story, after he just learned that he's essentially dying slowly. They know how to make him feel important, valued, and cared for. They know that is now their priority, not charting the assessment they just did on their last patient, or seeing if their coworker needs to go to lunch.

They're the nurses whose instincts all of the doctors trust.

They know how to make coworkers who hate each other, work together.

They know when they need to have a *come to Jesus meeting* when someone is in denial about the severity of the decisions they're making that are literally killing them. And they listen.

They are the ones with whom patients, families, and even coworkers feel comfortable being honest, even if it's painful and embarrassing.

They also know how to quickly grab control of a room full of frantic people when things start going downhill. They know how to convey urgency, not terror. They somehow make you feel safe when someone's life is literally a breath away.

Those nurses are my heroes. They're who I aspire to be every time I put my badge on in the morning. They're who I hope I have been when I clock out. They're the good nurses.

My prayer for you is that you become one of these nurses. These nurses not only save lives, but also profoundly affect each patient they touch with their blessed hands. My prayer for you is that you believe in yourself enough to do both the mental and emotional work to get there.

In saying that, it's hard to figure out how to be a good nurse when you're new. It feels like it's hopeless to get to the point of being a good nurse when you don't even know the first thing to do when your patient starts going downhill. When you look at the nurses that have been doing this for decades and think, "it'll take years and years before I get there," know that it doesn't have to. You can become a good, safe, efficient, and caring nurse without decades of experience behind you.

You just have to care.

You have to want to be better every day. Your patient has to be more important than your task list. What's better for your patient has to be more important than what's easier for you. You have to be willing to advocate for them when everyone is against you. You have to be willing to empathize, not sympathize, with your patient. It takes time to develop discernment in these situations, but you'll get there. You just have to *want* to get there.

The white of nursing is so very different from the black. It's much less straightforward and truly takes sitting with patients and their families in various situations to truly master it. You cannot learn this in a textbook. When you're brand new, you might not even realize how important this side of nursing is because you'll be so worried about just getting things done. Once you've been there for a patient who has an emotional break-down after getting more disappointing news, or when they're sad because no one visits, or once you've sat with a family right after the doctor told them their loved one is dying, you'll see that white side. Not that it'll get easier to be in that uncomfortable white space, but you'll get better at it.

And once you've seen and walked in that white side, you can blend to grey. You know when you need to just get everything done, but you also know which patients need extra time. You'll know how to support and educate a patient on getting a certain important test done that they've been refusing, but still get all of your meds passed and round with the physicians. You'll become the one that other nurses look to for guidance. Your wisdom will be undeniably calming. Your presence will put both coworkers and patience at ease. Your blend of nursing grey will be so glorious that before you know it, you'll become your unit's own Gandalf the Grey, BSN RN.

Everyone will be happy to see you're working on the same day as they are. You'll be able to handle any situation that may come your way with ease, confidence, and grace. You'll go from being a seemingly average person to the nurse that patients will never forget because you were there. You'll make Gandalf so proud that he'll come to your one hundred and eleven-tith birthday and set off the best fireworks display this side of the Shire.

And one of the beautiful things about nursing is some nurses are better at some things and some are better at others. A nursing unit is quite the team. I am somewhat of the emotional supporter on the team. I have some coworkers who are great at technical stuff (IV insertions, foley insertions, placing sutures, etc.), some who are great at having crucial conversations (calling a doctor back when they're not being responsive to patient's issue, pushing back to staffing when we need another nurse), and some who are great educators (can explain complicated medical conditions to people with the education of a 5th grader). It is really lovely to see a well-functioning unit work together, utilizing each other's strengths to best serve our patients.

Everyone blends to their own Gandalf Grey differently, with their own expertise in the mix. I've accepted that I won't be the best technical-skills nurse. I really come through for patients and loved ones with emotional needs.

I love when I'm working with my technical guy who has a calm demeanor, my crucial conversation nurse who calls anyone at the drop of a hat if we need something, my nurse who is basically an educator because she knows so much, and my motivated and proactive CNA. We're like the dream team. How safe would you feel if you knew a team of Gandalfs were manning the unit that your mom was on when she had a massive stroke?

No matter how crazy it gets, our patients are safe and expertly cared for. It's a beautiful thing. Each of us has had our own journey to blending to our Gandalf Grey (BSN RN) and becoming a good nurse. I know they're all good nurses and I respect and care for them like they're my family... my LOTR family.

CHAPTER 2

I'm a Survivor (of Nursing School)

I had absolutely no clinical experience prior to nursing school. Other than providing first aid to the kids who fell on the pool deck during my summers as lifeguard (despite telling them walk every 12 seconds), I had no experience being responsible for the care of another.

Therefore, my first clinical experience was utterly terrifying. I started getting nervous the week before. I tried to prepare as much as possible, but nothing could prepare me for what lay ahead.

Nursing school provides you with a lot of "firsts." I'd like to share with you two of my firsts —my first bed change and my very first assigned task in clinical.

You know how people say nothing can prepare you for children? Well, nothing can prepare you for your first experience changing a bedbound 300-lb patient who cannot move, and is covered in feces and urine in a small, non-ventilated nursing home room. Nothing.

My First Bed Change

Before I could begin real nursing clinicals, I had to become a certified nursing assistant (CNA). This meant completing nursing home clinicals, doing the down and dirty work. Feeding, bathing, and cleaning patients were the priority, something with which I had absolutely no experience.

Stop and think about the last time you were in a nursing home and take a full, deep breath of what you remember it smelling like.

...Did you do that yet?

Ugh. That.

My patient for the day was a large woman with advanced dementia. She could not speak or follow commands. She had lived in the nursing home for the past 10 years. Staff informed me that family rarely visited her. Basically, her life consisted of lying in bed and being turned and changed every few hours by the nursing staff. She was fed three meals a day by a nursing assistant. That was it. That was her life; quite the reality shock for my first day of clinicals.

Nevertheless, she was my patient for the day and I was going to take fantastic care of her... so I thought. As I came in to meet her for the first time, I smelled a smell I will never forget.

It was the very first time I had ever smelled feces mixed with urine. It made my eyes water. It's actually making my eyes water right now just thinking about it.

I left the room because I was in shock and had no idea what to do. Even though it may seem obvious what I needed to do, I had no idea how to actually go about doing it.

"How do you even move someone this large in this small of a bed to… you know… get all up in there?" I thought. I went to find my clinical instructor for what I thought was guidance but was actually just common sense.

"I think she has gone to the bathroom," I told my clinical instructor.

"Well, better go get some supplies and someone to help you clean her up!" she said and walked away.

I think all of the blood drained out of my face, and whatever I ate that morning for breakfast was flopping around in my stomach like Donald Trump's hairpiece on windy day.

So I grabbed what I thought I needed and found the first poor soul that I could find.

Thankfully, that poor soul was one of the nicest people in my nursing class. She was happy to help me, and I was ever so thankful.

We were both first-timers. The first time for me changing anyone in any capacity (no one in my family has babies so I'd never even changed a baby diaper at this point) and the first time for her changing an adult.

We looked at her like she was a puzzle, unsure of which piece to pick up first, as we tried to remember our simulation training. My classmate held the patient up on her side with all of her might in that tiny, poorly ventilated nursing home room to reveal the extent of the task that lay before me.

It was more than I could handle.

After I gagged 4-5 times while my classmate looked away so she didn't see it herself, I reluctantly began cleaning.

My eyes started to water as the smell of stool mixed with urine filled the room and our souls. I tried not to breathe at all, which clearly doesn't work for very long. I tried to breathe through my nose.

NOPE.

Dry heaves. Try something else.

Shallow breathing through my nose?

NOPE.

More dry heaves.

I'll try breathing through my mouth again.

NOPE.

I'm going to throw up. ABORT, ABORT!

I panicked because I didn't know how to breathe and not vomit on this poor woman.

I was trapped.

I profusely apologized to my classmate, who had started dripping sweat, and ran to the hallway for a taste of some sweet, sweet fresh air.

Nursing home air never smelled so good.

I took one last deep breath and ducked back in. We fumbled and struggled our way to get that woman squeaky clean.

Afterwards, I found my clinical instructor and had a breakdown moment. "I can't do this! I almost threw up doing the simplest thing a nurse can do!" I was almost in tears.

"You'll get used to it; it'll get better," my nursing instructor replied. I don't know if that was a deterrent, or comforting, but somehow I felt better.

The Man, the Student Nurse, and the Condom Catheter

As nursing school continued, things became more complex. Twice a week for eight hours, eight of my classmates and I met at a local hospital on their medical/surgical unit for our first real nursing clinical experience. Our first day, we were all very nervous. None of us knew what to expect.

Thankfully our clinical instructor was kind, hilarious, and a phenomenal teacher. We truly hit the jackpot. Once we were acclimated to the unit, she asked for a volunteer to complete a task. Determined to be an awesome student, I immediately volunteered.

"Great!" she excitedly said in front of the entire group. "We're going to go put a condom catheter on a male patient down the hall!"

"Um. Okay," I nervously replied. "I've never done that before. What do I need to do?" I was terrified and confused. I honestly couldn't even remember what a catheter was at that point.

As she showed us the condom catheter in her hand, I started to realize it was a little more straightforward than originally thought. "Well, have you ever put on a condom?" she loudly asked in front of all eight of my classmates that I just met the week prior.

With redness engulfing my face from embarrassment, I sheepishly replied, "no."

"Ugh. Already we're here. They already know too much about me," I thought as the judgments were forming. "She's either a prude or a slut," I assumed they were all thinking.

I wanted to just tell them all, "Hey guys, I'm one of those 'wait til you're married' type of girls," but thought day one of clinicals with people I met one week ago was just a little too soon. So, I just endured the stares and confused looks until my blushing face calmed back down to a terrified pale white.

I'm not sure if the extremely personal question even fazed her. After all, she was a nurse.

We walked into the room and there sat a 60-something year old man who looked like Santa—if he were completely bald, sunburnt, and angry. He was in a terrible mood. He had a stroke the day before and was having trouble doing anything he used to because he lost function on the left side of his body. And he was mad.

Something he was used to doing completely independently up until 24 hours ago was use the bathroom. Now he couldn't control it and kept urinating all over the bed. His skin became raw and the staff had to go through bed change after bed change. A condom catheter was the solution to his problem, but he wasn't too thrilled about it. They'd gone through about four of them because he just kept pulling them off because they didn't "fit right."

Well, guess who was about to reapply his fifth condom catheter? Yes, ladies and gentlemen... little old me on day one of clinicals.

Myself, my clinical instructor, and one other student headed in. My instructor explained what was about to happen, and he just grumbled in reply. He knew the drill. He knew he needed it, he just wasn't happy about it.

I put my gloves on, pulled the sheet back, and lifted his gown.

"You're going to feel cool down there," said my clinical instructor to the patient, who didn't seem to notice. She then instructed me to coat it with skin prep (something that makes the catheter stick to the penis) and then I rolled the condom catheter on.

Now, I don't mean to brag, but that catheter stayed on all day. A feat not conquered by any nurse previously. Nursing school is all about little victories and that man and his condom catheter were mine for the day.

I'll take what I can get.

Nursing School: Getting Through

Nursing school is all consuming. With frequent exams over hundreds of pages of material, multiple weekly clinicals, math exams, board reviews, and extensive pre-requisite requirements, you barely have time to ruin recipes you find on Pinterest anymore. Quite the tragedy, I know.

I'm what you call a typical B student. Not the top of my class, not the best test-taker, and woke up eight minutes before class every day. Not a slacker, but not trying to fight to the death for every single point, either. But after going through nursing school, I learned a few things.

Nursing school tests your patience, organization, graciousness, and dedication. You have to want it, you have to plan, and you have to focus on the big picture—becoming a nurse. And that means giving up and letting go of some things you may have worked hard for but may not be important in the long run.

I receive many questions about how to survive nursing school. I've narrowed them down to these Ten Nursing School Commandments.

Nurse Eye Roll's Ten Nursing School Commandments

1. **Thou Shalt Create A Calendar of Thy Assignments at the Beginning of the Semester.** Once you get all your syllabi (and recover from the subsequent myocardial infarction), get a calendar and write out all due dates for the entire semester. Plan when you will write your papers. Plan when you will study. Write out all of the exams, quizzes, and assignments on a calendar that you look at every day. That way you can wrap your head around everything and manage your time appropriately. I know it sounds crazy to plan when you will study a month or two out. However, there is such a large amount of information to know that a few hours the night before won't be enough to cut it. Be prepared, as Scar from *the Lion King* would say.

2. **Thou Shalt Work Smarter, and Harder.** I never wrote a paper the night before; I always finished at least five days in advance. I never stayed up all night to study; I was asleep by 2300 most nights before class. Frantically writing and studying last minute is an ineffective and inefficient use of time. Studying for six hours half asleep and exhausted is a waste of time. It would be more beneficial to you if you would focus and study for an entire hour using flashcards, re-typing your notes, going over them again and highlighting them, take a 30 minute break, and repeat for three total hours of studying. Be intentional with your time and plan how you will study. Don't just read from your textbook while falling asleep.

3. **Thou Shalt Make Time to Engage in Non-Nursing Activities and Spend Time With People Other Than Thy Classmates**. If you're all nursing all the time, only hanging out with people that only talk about nursing... you're going to go insane. And your family will get so sick of you talking about nursing that they'll go insane. Give yourself time away from the hectic life that is nursing school and de-stress. If you've managed your time appropriately, you won't have to stress about assignments whilst relaxing.

4. **Thou Shalt Not Care About What Your Classmates Got on Their Exams**. It's really easy after an exam to see what everyone else got. Don't. Try not to care about how others are doing. It'll only falsely inflate your ego, or if you're like me, make you feel bad about yourself because you didn't do as well. If you're not doing well, go chat with the professor on what you can do differently, not the girl next to you who gets 90 and above on every test and acts like it's no big deal. That'll just make you more frustrated and defeated every time you sit down to study.

5. **Thou Shalt Not Fight to the Death For Every Single Point**. On rare occasions it's worth it, but honestly... if you're mere points away from passing, something else is going on. Likewise, if you're someone getting great grades on all exams, don't waste everyone's time in class fighting about something that doesn't really make a difference, anyway. If you really care that much, speak with your professor privately. The stress that I saw a few points create for certain individuals during school was shocking. You can't win 'em all; you'll miss some points, even if you feel like you should have gotten something right. There will always be a question or two from left field that no one knows— just accept that it'll be there. Focus on passing, not on being the best. When you're at the bedside, no one cares what your GPA was. Put your heart and soul into understanding the information as a whole

and pass nursing school. If all you care about is a 4.0, you're doing it for the wrong reasons.

6. **Thou Shalt Not Engage in Drama With Classmates** Don't hook up with each other (awkward), don't complain to someone else about how this girl that annoys you always shows up late, or about what she wore to clinical that was totally unprofessional. That stuff can seem like a big deal in school, but honestly, it's not. Don't go complain to each other, don't create drama, and don't perpetuate it. Focus on what you need to do when you're there and don't care about what other people are or are not doing. It doesn't matter. You'll be annoyed at yourself three years later when you think about how much of your time and energy was spent talking about, entertaining, and perpetuating issues that didn't matter.

7. **Thou Shalt Attempt to Gain as Much Experience As Possible**. You learn procedures and skills by doing. So if you're kicking back in your clinicals, not volunteering to do things or letting your fear of the unknown keep you from stepping up to try things, you'll be screwed when you have to do it in the real world on your patient.

8. **Thou Shalt Take Care of Thyself**. Eat as healthy as your budget allows. Work out. Be sure to get adequate rest. If you're constantly drinking caffeinated soda to stay awake, eating junk food, and sleeping at odd times, it'll catch up with you. You'll gain weight and get depressed, and that my friend is a slippery slope. Even if you don't want to work out, make yourself. If you suffer from anxiety, depression, or something else, make sure you're addressing it appropriately and not waiting for it to become unbearable before you do something about it. Have the same expectations for yourself that you're going to have for your soon-to-be patients.

9. **Thou Shalt Familiarize Thyself with APA Style Writing and How to Obtain and Review Evidence-Based Research.** This will come up again and again, and the sooner you get it down and understand it, the faster you can write good papers and be done with them.

10. **Thou Shalt Take an NCLEX Review Course.** I took Kaplan. It provides you with a great paperback textbook, a lot of online resources, and makes studying for this as straight forward as possible.

Nursing school is not easy. It is a massive time commitment and tests you mentally, physically, and emotionally. It's hard, but it's worth it. Put in the time, work hard AND smart, make time for yourself to do non-nursing things, and just do the best you can with what you're given. This isn't one of those "just go through the motions" things. You have to try. You have to focus. There aren't shortcuts. And if you're slacking and trying to get by just doing the minimum, I don't want you to be my nurse.

Studying the Right Way

A lot of your time will be spent studying. As I said in my commandments, be intentional with your time. Falling asleep while reading for five hours doesn't count. So no, you can't go complain to people that you stayed up super late studying and didn't even pass your exam.

Be effective in your studying. Different courses require different approaches. For example, pharmacology requires straightforward memorization. Flashcards are best. Also, make up hilarious and unforgettable associations to remember certain terms, meds, conditions, etc. Many times during exams, I could be seen laughing to myself because of some absurd thing I came up with to remember something.

For those exams that are not so straightforward but are over hundreds of pages of material, your approach should be different. You want to understand the concept as a whole so that you can appropriately answer questions. For example, don't memorize seemingly important sentences about heart failure. That doesn't help you put the entire picture together. Learn about heart failure as a whole and try to explain it to someone. That is way more valuable and memorable than six hours of reading. Furthermore, you'll be able to field questions that aren't verbatim from the text.

Figure out how you learn best. Personally, I would take notes in class and then go home and type them. That meant I was going over them at least twice. And then at the end of the semester when we had our comprehensive finals, I'd have all of my notes typed and organized to reference. Some classmates would record the lectures and listen to them again when they were driving. That didn't work so much for myself (I'd just think of other things) but it did work well for others.

Don't over-highlight. I know you want to highlight everything, but that's just like highlighting nothing. If everything is important, the basically nothing is important. Only highlight the essential things.

Something that always seemed to get me was forgetting to read the captions the pictures of my textbooks. There was always a question that came from one of those that had information that was nowhere else in the text. Don't forget about the captions!

Furthermore, I highly recommend doing an internship during the summer. It is extremely beneficial for practical knowledge but can also help you get a job after graduation. During the summer between my junior and senior years of nursing school, I was accepted into a nursing internship at a large local hospital. It was an invaluable experience and helped me land my first job.

As an intern, you get exposed to so many things that get you comfortable with the environment and it really puts you a step ahead of other applicants. Nurses, CNA's, and nurse managers know your name and you get familiar with the flow of everything. Seriously guys, if you have an opportunity to do this (paid or not), I highly recommend applying for one of these in the early months of your spring semester of your junior year. In this market it's tough for new grads to get a job. You need anything that'll give you an edge. This was my edge.

Entrapment: Nobody Puts Baby in a Corner

I completed my internship on a 40-bed surgical floor that had about 10 step-down rooms. My preceptor and myself were caring for a 650lb male patient in his early 30s in one of the step-down rooms.

Patients of this weight have very specific needs to complete routine care. They need a bed much larger and stronger than regular beds to support their size and weight. They have to be in a room with a door that opens wider than normal doors. They have to have an extra-large bedside commode to support their weight and the width of their backside. These patients are almost always bed bound because their knees and feet cannot support their weight.

Typically when someone weighs this much, it's hard to breathe. These patients usually have problems breathing for two main reasons. One, their necks are so large that they cannot keep their airway open, and often times need a *tracheostomy* to breathe through. Second, the sheer weight of their chest prevents their lungs from expanding properly. This patient had both of these issues during this admission.

> *Nurse-ipedia Definition: A tracheostomy (trach) is a surgically created hole in the neck that allows someone to*

breathe. They're inserted so we can always maintain their
airway and provide adequate oxygenation.

He was admitted for hypoxia (low oxygen) due to extreme morbid obesity and was on a *ventilator,* which was connected to his *tracheostomy* (because he couldn't maintain his own airway) when he first arrived. He had graduated to a point where he just needed the tracheostomy and no longer needed the machine.

> **Nurse-ipedia Definition:** *A ventilator (vent) is a machine*
> *that breathes for the patient. When someone is on one, we*
> *say they're "vented."*

He had already coded twice during this admission.

My preceptor came to let me know the patient told him that he needed to have a bowel movement. My eyes widened with disbelief and concern. In the busyness of the day, it had never occurred to me to think about what we would have to do if he had to have a bowel movement.

My preceptor explained to me that we had to get him up to the bedside commode.

Again, my eyebrows furrowed with confusion. The mechanics of it boggled my mind.

"How on earth are we going to do this?" I thought, as my preceptor started walking around the unit, recruiting nurses to help us complete this seemingly impossible task.

It was going to take seven of us to get this man to go from his bed, which was half the width of the room, to the bedside commode, which was a fourth of the width of the room. We also grabbed a couple of physical therapists, a tech, and a few nurses. This was going to be quite a feat.

We gathered supplies to change his bed, as we had to take advantage of the time that he would be out of the bed. We were going to clean the bed that he'd been sitting on for his entire admission. We had been rolling him side to side to clean him and the bed, but needed to do a deep clean while we could. We were also planning on cleaning in between various folds of his skin that were previously inaccessible with him in the bed. Nurses really know how to maximize their time.

At 650lbs, each extremity weighed about the same as each staff member. We sat him up with one manning each leg, two at his back, and one on each arm with an additional person standing by just in case. This alone caused us all to begin to perspire.

We shuffled him to the edge of the bed with the help of a solid sheet and good ergonomics. Miraculously, he was able to stand with the support of a bariatric walker.

In the frantic shuffle of things, somehow I got pinned between the wall and the commode. As I slowly put the pieces of the situation together, I came to a realization.

My position in the room could only mean one thing: I was the only one who would be able to wipe his backside when he was done. Me.

(Gulp) "I can do this. I can do this," I thought as I put on my eye-of-the-tiger face. I gave myself a mini-pep talk. I took a few deep breaths to get my mind right. "This is going to happen whether I like it or not, so I better make it count. This is going to be the best tush-wiping I've ever done," I thought.

If it wasn't completely unprofessional, I would have slowly made eye contact with everyone in the room and confidently said, "Bring it on," like we were down 20 points at halftime and were ready to destroy our opponent with cleanliness.

Now, in case you didn't know, if you have a tracheostomy, you cannot talk without a special valve. This patient had the trach but had not advanced to the point where he could have the valve to talk to us. Communication consisted of gestures and a dry-erase white board.

As you can imagine, he was pretty tuckered out just from standing up. He shuffled the three steps to get himself positioned to where he needed to be in front of the commode. We anticipated that this would be exhausting for him and we all paused with him to allow him a moment to rest.

There I stood, pinned against the wall, waiting for him to sit down. I watched everything unfold from my helpless position. Nurses were on both sides of him, and in front guiding and supporting him to where he needed to be.

Even from behind him, unable to see his face, I could tell he was exhausted. This was the most movement and exercise he had gotten in weeks. He was breathing pretty heavily.

He started leaning forward on his walker, seemingly doing so to catch his breath. My eyes widened as all of the dramatic worst-case scenarios started running through my mind. "If he codes and falls, three nurses will break their legs and we'll never get him back into a bed," I thought.

Once he had himself secured against the walker, I heard it. I heard it being birthed from depths of his bowels. It was a fart, and it was coming my way. Fast.

A tiny one sneaked out. Then, the feature presentation began. It was loud. It was musical. And it lasted a lot longer than anyone was prepared to endure.

I immediately started "shallow nurse breathing" so as not to deeply breathe in the terrible, gut-wrenching odors and subsequently lose what little nourishment I had previously consumed on the sanitized hospital floor (a skill quickly developed in nursing school).

My eyebrows raised and my eyes started to water. There was no escape; I was in the thick of it until we crossed the finish line.

When he started to back towards the commode, he turned his head and I saw him sneak out a smile. A kind of, "whoops – got ya!" smile. Not that he did it on purpose, but could clearly find the humor in this crazy situation that I'm sure he never pictured himself in.

I slowly turned and looked to my coworkers who were all barely holding in laughter as they all were looking in different corners of the room. They were doing the same shallow nurse breathing, trying not to make eye contact with one another, afraid that if we did we would all lose control and erupt into an untamable, infectious burst of laughter.

Don't get me wrong, nurses have phenomenal poker faces. The best of the best. But when a 650lb man slowly bends over and, without warning, passes gas in the face of an innocent and naïve 21-year old nursing student trapped in the corner, —all bets are off.

I know we all sound insensitive at this particularly sensitive moment in this patient's life, but the reason we were all trying so hard not to laugh is because we didn't want the patient to feel embarrassed. I know he was smiling, but it was still important to maintain composure. In a normal day, we get about as up close and personal as it gets, and we have learned to keep a straight face through even the most ridiculous of circumstances.

We were trying to maintain his dignity, and darn it, we succeeded. Not one person laughed aloud. Everyone was calm and supportive. I was pretty impressed with the entire team in that moment. We kept it together and got him on the commode. He was very thankful for our efforts and we were thankful for his.

A few of us stayed in the room with him while he attempted to go. I, of course, being pinned to the wall, had to stay. A few of the nurses winked at me with grins on their faces as they walked out of the room.

Twenty minutes passed. Nothing.

After all of that, he couldn't go. We got him back in bed the same way we had gotten him out. Fartless this time.

I slowly walked to the nurse's station in silence and sat down to reflect on the events that had just transpired.

Quietly I sat. And reflected.

"Did that just happen?" I asked the nurse charting next to me who was unfazed by everything.

Without hesitation she replied, "Welcome to nursing." She smiled and immediately returned to her charting.

I heard a call light go off. It was his. He had bowel movement in the bed.

As I walked into the room with supplies in my hand, he had a big grin on his face and mouthed "oops!" to me.

Seriously, welcome to nursing!

Passing the NCLEX

After you get done with your classes and clinicals, walk across the stage, and go through your pinning ceremony, you still have to pass boards. Yes, you have your degree but it doesn't mean much without being licensed.

It's pretty overwhelming when years of grueling schoolwork culminate to one terrifying exam.

There's no way to completely take the stress out of this ridiculous process, but I think if you approach it with intention, you can reduce the amount of stress significantly. And don't listen to those people who are fabulous test-takers who say prep courses are a waste of money and just bought a $20 book, studied for a night, took it hung-over, and passed. They're the exception, not the rule.

I'll tell you a little bit about my post-graduation timeline. I graduated in May and took a full week off after graduation and didn't look at one text-book or think about nursing at all. 'Twas glorious. You desperately need this break after nursing school. For your sanity, please take some time off.

After one of the best weeks of my life, I took the week-long Kaplan Review Course the third week of May. I highly, highly recommend this course.

When Kaplan started, I put all of my nursing books from school away (honestly, I've barely looked at them since) and focused on the book that Kaplan gave me. I did what they told me during the course and followed their plan.

I didn't cross reference things from various books, I didn't buy an NCLEX study guide, I didn't cram, and I didn't try to read as much as possible. It's just too much information. You should already have a general knowledge base; now you just need to know how to break the questions down to get to the answer. Yes, there will be some knowledge-based things you don't know, but the Kaplan book provides the knowledge you'll need in addition to test-taking skills. I really liked that book because it was concise yet comprehensive so I didn't feel like I needed to look at other books to study appropriately.

I did the recommended 25-50 questions daily for 4 weeks until I sat for boards. I took one day off per week of no questions or studying (again, sanity preservation). I do not recommend waiting months to sit for boards. The longer you wait, the more you forget. Just get the test over and done.

I took my test three hours away in the afternoon the second week of June. I got great sleep the night before, had my husband drive me so I could relax on the way, and also had him take me out to lunch right before. I definitely had a delicious beer with lunch. I think that helped with my nerves.

I was done in 1 hour and 15 minutes and passed with 75 questions.

Reminder: I'm not a 4.0 student and not a great test-taker.

You will walk out feeling like you failed, with symptoms of diarrhea, nausea, and vomiting. You'll feel like that even if you graduated Summa Cum Laude and are a great test-taker. You just spent years fighting for every single point, all while getting used to an 80% needed to pass, however the NCLEX is structured very differently than nursing school exams. The percentage needed to pass the NCLEX is much lower than that. If you look it up online, they break down the scoring in depth. They also go over it in review courses, which is another reason to take one!

I know nurses who timed-out after the six allotted hours and passed. I know those who got all 265 questions and passed in three hours. I know quite a few who passed in 75-120 questions. I know one who passed with 75 questions in 20 minutes.

Pick a study course and stick to it, take days off, test as soon as you're ready, and relax the day before.

If you don't pass the first time, figure out what you need to do the second time around. The world is not over if you didn't pass. I know multiple amazing nurses who did not pass their first time. That test does not define your career. I've never had any patient or family member ask me how many times I took my boards. I've also never had a job application ask for that information.

If you didn't do a review course, now is the time. You must be disciplined, do what they recommend, and focus. No excuses, no short cuts.

Coming Around Full Nursey Circle

You won't put together the picture you're painting of what it means to be a nurse until you're a few years into your career. You get bits and pieces in school, trying to make sense of it all as you plug along with assignments, clinicals, and many firsts. Your first bed change, your first IV start, your first foley insertion on a morbidly obese, confused, and combative female patient with odd anatomy, your first code, your first death, and the first time a patient at death's door comes back to the unit months later completely healthy to tell you thank you for caring for them during the worst time in their life.

Once you start to walk through these experiences, your picture of nursing will become clearer. You'll be able to understand things on a deeper level. Your critical thinking skills will develop and become more comprehensive. You'll master the basics and therefore won't have to stress about them anymore.

Things that seem impossible at the beginning are suddenly not only possible, but easy. Things that you thought would take an hour, take at most three minutes. Things that you thought would make you vomit don't all of a sudden. And not only that, you can go to lunch minutes later and still enjoy your meal just the same.

Nursing presents so many challenges to you. Challenges you never though you'd be able to conquer. So when you're in school and think there's no way this can get any easier, hold on to the hope that it will.

Before, I was terrified to turn and clean that nursing home patient. I almost threw up! Now I can clock-in with confidence, knowing I can handle most situations that will come my way and know who to call for the situations in which I am clueless.

Those first few experiences molded who I am as nurse. That poopy bed change and that huge fart were just the beginning of this crazy nursing journey. Oddly enough, I am thankful for those experiences. And thankful and amazed that God has graced me with the desire and the joy to continue.

CHAPTER 3

Graduate Nurse Turned Bedside Nurse

===

Once you graduate from nursing school and pass your boards, you'll be flung into the "real world" of nursing. The theoretically perfect hospital that you've based all of your learning off of does not exist. There are many barriers between doing things the textbook-correct way, and the way it's really done in practice. You're missing supplies, you're short staffed, your patient/family isn't agreeable or compliant, the doctor won't answer pages, your coworkers are not helpful, the people you delegate to give you attitude and won't complete whatever task that's been delegated to them.

There are all of these very real barriers that occur, and you're never taught how to deal with them. And guess when you'll have to deal with them all at once for the first time…your very first day as a bedside nurse! The overwhelming feelings of, "I can't handle this" and, "I was not prepared for this," settle in.

Now, I'm not saying these things always happen, but occasionally they do. You're expected to deal with it, as Katie Duke would say, and figure out how to get done what you need to get done for your patients.

This huge gap between our supposed college preparedness and how to do our actual job is left for the hospitals to fill. The hospitals are always slashing their budgets, and looking for ways to save. One of the first things to change is the way nursing care is delivered. Working with the minimum is the name of the game, so those of us new graduates who don't have a clue either sink or swim during our first few months.

It's a cold, nursey world out there.

But don't give up hope! What you are feeling is normal. Simply continue on. Once you get past this point, the sun shines down on you like the first day of spring. It is so rewarding, you would think you have a reward's card on your keychain that you swipe each time a tearful elderly woman thanks you for caring for her confused husband.

Now before I get into the nitty-gritty of it, I want to shortly talk about landing a nursing job.

Landing a Job

The market is tough right now. Hospital budgets are slim, and something they have to be selective about is which nurses they hire. This means it is harder for new nurses to get jobs because they don't yet have experience.

New graduates have to work hard to stand out. Here's my list of things that jump out to recruiters:

1. **A bachelor's degree in nursing (BSN):** A lot of hospitals are going to start looking at that as a requirement (and if you have an ADN, have a plan to obtain your BSN within a certain amount of time).

2. **Experience at that particular hospital/facility:** Maybe you were a CNA, a phlebotomist, or a secretary at that facility. If you're already

familiar with it, there's less of a learning curve, and there are people they can directly contact within the system to see what kind of impression you've left.

3. **Volunteer experience:** You've taken time out of your busy nursing school schedule to help out others. Major bonus points.

4. **References other than your nursing school professors:** The more people you have on your team, the better. Everyone from your nursing class will have their professors on their resume. Who else knows you're awesome? Who else will vouch for you?

5. **Phenomenal letters of recommendation:** I had one of the physicians I worked with in nursing school write a letter of recommendation for me. I also volunteered at a hospital and had the volunteer services coordinator write me a recommendation. I know it can be scary to ask these people, but it can make a huge difference.

Getting the call for the interview is step one. Step two is rocking the interview. Nursing recruiters base a lot on interviews. You're going to be at the front lines of their company, and they want to make sure you have great interpersonal skills. Therefore, you rocking that interview is essential. Here are some of my hints to landing the job.

RN Job Interviews

1. **Make a good impression with the person at the front desk.** Many times, interviewers ask the front desk person what their impression was. They know you'll be on your best behavior at the interview, but they want to see what kind of impression you left on everyone. Be nice and don't talk or complain loudly on the phone for all to hear while you wait.

2. **Look GOOD.** Professional, put together, organized. Have one of those leather portfolios with a resume <u>printed on resume paper</u>. They'll already have one, but give them a "fresh one" when you sit down. And make sure your resume is perfect. There are a lot of helpful websites out there that talk about building the perfect resume. Do some research and perfect your resume!

3. **Know the hospital's mission statement, vision, and values, and work it into the conversation.** Talking about this shows the recruiter that you have done your homework. You've put in the time. Take a look at it online and relate your work ethic and/or values to theirs. Talk about how you will make a great fit because of this.

4. **Practice answering a few questions beforehand:** They'll ask you about patient experiences, so make sure you have some fresh in your brain before the interview begins. They can be hard to remember during interviews because it all just blurs together and that's why I'm a big fan of going through a practice round of questions with a close friend or two. For example, think about a time you went above and beyond, a time you handled a tough situation well, and a time you could have handled things differently, etc. Always be ready for the "why did you go into nursing" question, and have a real answer. And it's okay to have things written down in your professional leather portfolio. You look prepared.

5. **Be prepared for the "3 weaknesses and 3 strengths" question, and have real answers for the weaknesses.** They know the whole "too detailed, caring too much, working too hard" thing is just regurgitated information. Again, have real and honest answers.

6. **Be prepared with questions for them.** You should always have quality questions. Below are some examples.

- What kind of a clinical ladder, if any, do you have?

- You should know if they're a Magnet hospital or not. If they are, ask when they were designated and about their Magnet journey. If they are not, ask if they are working on obtaining their designation.

- What percent of your nurses are nationally certified?

- What is the average nurse-to-patient ratio? Has the average changed recently?

- What's your average length of orientation for new grads?

- Is there a transition program for graduate nurses becoming bedside nurses?

- If/when I decide to work on my master's, do you offer any assistance and do you work closely with any nearby nursing schools?

- Is nursing incivility a problem on your unit?

- Tell me about the culture of safety on the unit.. (by this I mean, if there is a fall on a unit, how it that handled? Do they have a reporting system? Are the employees themselves concerned about safety and therefore ensure all precautions are being taken consistently? Or, is the culture more of a "do it the easiest and quickest way even if it's not safe" culture?).

- How involved is your unit in Shared Governance?

- Is there anything about my application that concerns you?

7. **Follow up with a handwritten thank you note.** If you didn't interview with the actual nurse manager you'd be working under, make

sure you get a business card from the person who interviewed you. If you didn't do that, ask the person at the front desk or call and ask later. Send one to every single person who interviewed you. Again, you will stand out and be memorable.

Example: *"Thank you so much for taking the time to interview me for the open nursing position on your _____ unit. I enjoyed meeting you and learning about you and your team. I appreciate your time and consideration. After getting to know you and learning more about the unit, I believe I would make an excellent addition to your team. I believe that my _____, _____, and _____ make me a perfect candidate. Feel free to contact me with any additional questions. Again, thank you for your time and consideration."*

8. **Know that they'll Google you, look at your Facebook, Twitter, Instagram, etc.** Google yourself before you even begin applying. Anything you don't want a potential employer seeing, take it down. I am not joking here, guys. They will Google you and will use that as a reason not to hire you. Drunk college pics, controversial posts, sexual stuff… it all tells the world, including potential employers, what kind of a person you are. The whole MTV Scrubbing In show is a prime example. We don't work in just any field. People's lives will be in your hands and you don't want to give potential employers a reason not to want you representing their company. You are in one of the most trusted professions in America, dealing with sensitive patient information. Because of this, you are held to a higher standard. Be smart when it comes to posting things on social media, and research yourself.

If you're thinking, "I don't need to do all of that, I'll just go in and be myself and if they don't like me then I'll just work somewhere that does." **UM, NO.** It's difficult for even experienced RN's to land a job; so new grads need to be on top of their game in interviews. Do all the little stuff so you actually get an offer and start working and getting paid, like, now.

So Now That You Have a Job...

I was blessed enough to have an amazing preceptor and a really good new graduate residency program straight out of nursing school. I felt very supported by my preceptor, my manager, and the educators running the residency program. Myself and the 40 other new grads met together once a week for four hours to discuss our progress and to have various leaders of the hospital come through and discuss their roles and just get us familiarized with the culture of the hospital. Seriously, every hospital needs a program like this. Nursing satisfaction goes up, turnover goes down. It's a beautiful thing.

Calling Doctors

My preceptor was only a few years older than me and had been a nurse on our cardiovascular and thoracic surgical step-down for about three years. I looked at her with awe and wonder. She knew everything. Everyone knew her. Patients responded well to her. She got done on time. My goal was to be like her.

Over the course of three months, she slowly molded me as a nurse. She showed me how to do the thing in which I was most uncomfortable: calling doctors. In nursing school, doctors don't want to talk to nursing students. They want to talk to the nurse, get the information they need, and move on. Therefore, upon graduation from school, many nurses have never paged a physician before. The first time I paged one I almost had a panic attack. I didn't know what they'd want, what questions they'd ask, or if they'd be mean like they were in all of the horror stories my coworkers would tell. I had my preceptor right there almost literally holding my hand. It was the best I could do to not pee on myself.

For those of you that are equally as terrified, I came up with some helpful hints on how to approach this daunting task.

1. **Don't immediately apologize for calling them.** Yes, it sucks you had to bother them, but it's their job and you're just doing yours. It's all business.

2. **Don't get nervous and just say the patient's name and ask your question.** You could be talking to an on-call doctor who may not be familiar with your patient, or they may need a few key pieces of information to jog their memory on this patient. If you're not sure, first ask if they are familiar with your patient. If they're not, give them a <u>brief</u> summary of the patient's main problems. Physicians see a long list of patients and may need a little reminding of what Mr. Brown came in with six days ago.

3. **Don't refer to your patient as their room number.** For some reason, nurses refer to patients as their room number (probably because of multiple admissions, discharges, and transfer during one shift). Typically, inpatient physicians see their patients during their entire admission and follow them from room to room; therefore they always refer to them by their name. So if you call and say, "Hi Dr. Patel, I'm calling about the patient in room 872." They will always say, "And who would that be?" This also isn't a good habit for nurses to get into, anyway. Try to refer to your patient by their name, and not their room number, throughout the shift.

4. **Be prepared.** Have a fresh set of vitals, know their allergies, have their labs pulled up, anticipate their questions, and be in a quiet area

because half the time I swear I can barely hear them because they're whispering. It's like I'm calling them in the middle of mass or something. If possible, know what order you want. For example, if they've had an increase in premature ventricular contractions (PVC's) and have had a lot of urinary output, anticipate that they may want to check labs. If they're hypotensive with no fluids running and minimal oral intake, anticipate a fluid bolus. Try to know what you want before you call.

5. **If it's a recurring problem, ask when they want to be notified again.** If you're calling because they had a three second pause and their heart rate is in the 40s and he tells you he doesn't care, ask when he wants to be notified and have an order that reflects that. There's no reason to constantly interrupt their day (or yours!).

6. **Make sure you have scratch paper handy to write down orders.** You think you'll remember it, but then he or she gives you four unexpected med orders and your CNA is trying to talk to you while you're on the phone and now you've forgotten them all before you've hung up. And if you work somewhere that requires you to stay on the phone with them while entering orders, know that doesn't always happen. Sometimes they're in a hurry, in the car, in surgery, or dealing with another very real emergency and don't have the time for you to slowly enter a non-emergent order. Be ready to quickly write something down if needed.

7. **Don't page and go do something else.** Nothing makes them more upset than being paged, then waiting on hold while you finish getting someone off the bedpan for 12 minutes. I think I would be frustrated, too! Catch up on some charting or be near the desk when you page. However, if it's been over 20 minutes, page again.

8. **Ask your fellow RN's if they also need to speak with that doctor.** Address all of your needs simultaneously so that you're not continuing to interrupt the physician while they're seeing other patients. This will also save your coworkers some time as well; they won't have to stop what they're doing to page and wait if they know you're about to page the physician.

9. **If they're rude, don't take it personally.** The sooner you accept that, the better. Doctors get mad and rude sometimes, but that doesn't have to make you feel like crap for the rest of the shift. Maybe they had a patient they had been heavily invested in die earlier that day, maybe their kid won't stop crying and he had just fallen asleep, or maybe they're just awful. Regardless of what's going on during their day, there is no reason for them to be disrespectful to you. You need to be confident and secure enough with yourself to know that if they're being rude, it's not always about you. Deal with it appropriately (whether it be firmly telling them not to speak to you like that or letting your manager know) and go on with the rest of your day. Their negative attitude does not get to steal your joy from you all day. It just doesn't.

So, how do you go about doing this, you ask?

Example of How Confident and Awesome You Will Be..

RING RING!! RING RING!!

"This is Dr. Smith."

"Hi Dr. Smith, this is Jaclyn Evans from the stroke floor. I have a question about the patient Edward Godwin in room 8123. Are you familiar with him?"

"No. My partner admitted him overnight and I've yet to round on him."

"He came in yesterday for a left thalamic ischemic stroke. He did not receive tPA on admission. At baseline, he has right-sided weakness and numbness/tingling. Otherwise, he's been alert and oriented all day. I'm calling because he's really difficult to wake up. Before, even when sleeping, he would awaken appropriately for staff. Now, I practically have to do a sternal rub to get him to follow commands."

"What was his sodium this morning and how have blood pressures been running?"

"Sodium was 131 and it looks like he has voided approximately 5 liters in the last six hours. His latest blood pressure is 117/68. His systolic tends to run 120-140."

"Is he protecting his airway?"

"He's started snoring, which is new, but otherwise he's been 100% on room air."

"Get a STAT head CT scan and I'm going to transfer him to intensive care. Hopefully you can just take him straight there after the scan. You may want to call your rapid response team to assist you in case he becomes unstable."

"Ok thanks!"

Orders you would anticipate:

STAT BMP

STAT head CT without contrast

Transfer to a higher level of care

Note: if you are transferring your patient to a higher level of care, you must take the patient yourself to the receiving unit. That is the safest thing to do with a patient that is decompensating.

Rounding with Physicians

I also want to talk a little bit about rounding with physicians. Try to round with them as they see your patients. It's not always possible, but when you're able to do this, it is very beneficial.

If you round with the doctors, you can consolidate your needs and concerns all at once while they're with the patient. Every morning when I get report, I make a list of the things I need to clarify with the physician. I don't immediately page them when I find out that I have a non-urgent need. Many things, if not most, can wait until the physician is rounding.

This is also important because you're talking to them when they are focused on your patient. They are at your patient's bedside; they didn't have to stop what they were doing with another patient to refocus on yours. Now, I'm not saying never page the doctors. When you need them, page them. However, if you have multiple non-emergent needs that will not change the immediate care of the patient or just need to clarify something, make everyone's life easier and just wait for them to round.

However, keep an eye on the time. If I notice it's 1600 and I know the on-call doctor starts at 1700 and I've been waiting all day to touch base with this particular physician, I'll go ahead and page them. I want to make sure they'll see the patient before they go off for the night. If they won't be coming by for some reason, then I get all of my questions and/or needs addressed on the phone at that time.

Which Doctor Are You Again?

Something else people didn't explain to me was the difference between an attending physician, consulting physician, and physician's assistant/nurse practitioner.

Here's how it works:

Whatever doctor decides to admit the patient is called the attending physician. This person is in charge; they ultimately call the shots (ha!). Typically this is a hospitalist or internal medicine physician. However, if a patient was admitted for a particular surgery, that surgeon is the attending. (For example, if they get admitted for a brain tumor that needs to be removed, the neurosurgeon will be the attending. If the patient is admitted and needs a coronary artery bypass graft, the cardiovascular surgeon will be the attending.)

As this attending physician deems necessary, they will consult physicians from other service lines. (Examples of service lines include neurology, nephrology, general surgery, cardiology, etc.) So, if the patient was admitted for a brain tumor by a neurosurgeon, but the patient has a bunch of comorbidities (additional health problems), they most likely will consult the internal medicine team to manage those issues so they can focus on the management of the brain tumor.

Let me give you an example..

A patient is admitted with severe leg pain. After performing appropriate diagnostics in the emergency room, it was determined that the patient will need to have a femoral-popliteal bypass. The cardiovascular surgeon admits the patient and plans to operate tomorrow. However, this patient takes many medications for his uncontrolled hypertension and he is in acute renal failure. The cardiovascular surgeon (the attending doctor) decides to consult the hospitalist for medical management (the consulting physician). After surgery, the patient's condition declines, needs dialysis, has been noted to flip in and out of uncontrolled atrial fibrillation and despite starting Cardizem, he continues to have an uncontrolled heart rate. After speaking with the cardiovascular surgeon (attending), the hospitalist decides to consult nephrology to manage his renal failure as well as cardiology to manage his cardiac issues. Again, the cardiovascular surgeon remains the attending physician, while the hospitalist, nephrologist, and cardiologist are all consulting physicians. However, when a patient begins to have complex medical issues after a surgery, occasionally the surgeon will ask the medical physician to take over as the attending physician.

Typically most physicians have a nurse practitioner (NP) and/or physician assistant (PA) who works with them. They do a lot of legwork for the physicians. I love them dearly. They will deal with most day-to-day issues. I almost always call the NP/PA first if they have one. If it's something I need to speak directly to the MD about, they'll either communicate it to them or tell me to page them myself. These instances are the exception and not the rule. The NP/PA typically can handle most issues that may arise.

When you're trying to figure out which physician to call, you need to think critically for a moment. If there are multiple physicians consulted and you're not sure, think about which service is the most appropriate to address the problem. If it's a question about insulin and a surgeon is the attending but medicine is consulted, I'd call the medicine physician or NP/PA. If a medical doctor is the attending but you have a question about orders for surgery in the morning, I'd call the surgeon's NP/PA.

If you have a question about a specific order, check to see which physician ordered it originally.

Report

Ah, *report*. Every unit does it a little differently. Learning how to give an efficient, concise yet detailed report is part of being a good nurse.

> **Nurse-ipedia definition:** *Report is the time when nurses are switching shifts and pass information to each other about the plan of care for each patient.*

I love it when someone is good at giving report. They communicate appropriately, clock out on time, and I can get started early. We all win.

Elements of a good report:

1. **t's systematic.** You go through it the same way every single time. You always start with name, age, code status, doctors, and allergies and you end with clarifying questions for the rounding physician. You go through each pertinent body system one at a time. If it's not systematic, typically information is omitted.

2. **It's informative but not unnecessarily detailed.** I want to know the things about this patient that are pertinent to the next 12 hours and their overall admission. I want you to tell me the abnormals. I don't think you're a bad nurse if your report is short and concise.

3. **It quickly tells me how they got to be on our unit, what we're doing for them, our plan of care, and any emotional considerations.** I want big-picture things that I can't quickly pick out from the chart. While it's nice to know their IV access, what fluids are running, and if they're wearing SCD's or not, I can already see all of that on the chart. I also like to ask the off going nurse if the patient and family are doing okay emotionally. I like to get a feel of the emotional climate of the

room before I go in and know about important conversations that have occurred.

4. **No one interrupts.** When I get report, I don't ask questions until the end. If someone asks me a question, I say, "Hold on until I'm done and I'll answer it," because I almost always was going to address that already. If someone is giving you report, do not go through your report sheet asking them questions in the order in which you want to receive information. That is not how report flows. The reporting nurse tells you about the patient and you ask clarifying questions afterwards.

5. **It's considerate.** Do not spend the first 10 minutes of designated report looking up information on your patients. Be considerate of other people's time. They've been here the last 12 hours; please don't make them wait because you want to look up information. If you want to know about your patient before report, you need to arrive early. Similarly, manage your time at the end of your shift so that you're not in a room doing something else you could have done earlier when report needs to get started.

Futhermore, I recommend keeping the same report sheet for three to four shifts before tossing it and trying a different format. I tried about three before I finalized the one I like. I have it memorized, and because of that, I typically can give report completely off the top of my head and not forget anything because I can mentally go through the sheet.

Assessments

I took an assessment class in nursing school. It wasn't anything like what I do in the real nursing world.

It was way too broad and vastly different for each specialty that they wanted to insure we experienced. Don't get me wrong, I'm glad I saw the

OR, OB, mental health, the ED, the ICU, and various floors, but one thing that I didn't get out of all of that was solid practical assessment skills for a normal floor patient.

Here's how to quickly rock a basic assessment for a basic med-surg floor patient.

(Keep in mind this is <u>basic</u>. If you work in a specialized area, this assessment would be insufficient. Please refer to your unit's standards.)

Talk to them.
What's your name? What year is it? Do you know where you are right now? How'd you get to be with me here in the hospital?

This normal convo tells you a lot about their neurological status. It'll tell you if they're alert and oriented, if their speech is clear, and if their face is symmetrical when they talk. Don't just chitchat with them; ask them specific questions to assess their orientation status. Some patients can seem like they're really with it, and then you ask them what year it is and they say, "Why, it's 1921, of course!" I always tell them to humor me as I ask my silly questions, as to not insult anyone or throw them off, and proceed to ask them their name, the location, why they're in the hospital, and the month/year.

Walk around their bed, see if they focus on you and track you appropriately as well.

Shine a pen light in their eye.
Are their pupils equal, do they react briskly, and do they accommodate light appropriately?

Listen.

Listen to their lungs in six spots on their back, then their heart in three to four spots, then their bowel sounds in all four quadrants. Start listening in the right lower quad, which is where the ileocccecal valve, and therefore loudest bowel sounds, is located.

Ask when their last bowel movement was. If it was within the last 24 hours, ask if it was loose/diarrhea. Most patients are on some sort of stool softener, so this will tell you if you need to hold it or not. However, if they are taking pain meds or are fresh post op, make sure they get their stool softener!

Palpate their abdomen; ask if there is any abdominal pain and note if it is distended or firm.

Grip and feel.

Have them grip your hands and let go on command a few times and do a good push/pull, then feel their radial pulses. Have them hold out their hands, palms up, with their eyes closed for 10 seconds to check for a drift.

Dorsi/plantar flexion and feel.

Have them dorsi/plantar flex on your hands and then feel their pedal pulses.

If you don't know where those are, I'm sure your assessment textbook over-explains it somewhere.

Ask questions.

Are you having any numbness/tingling? (Sensory assessment.) If they say yes, are diabetic, have a history of neuropathy, and always have numbness/tingling, ask if it is different than normal.

Are you in pain? Please rate it on a scale of 1-10. Don't forget to tell them that a 10 is burning alive or being eaten by a bear or something.

Do you have any questions about our plan today or anything you want to ask the doctor? This is just to make sure you're on the same page about what's going on.

Assess the skin.

It is essential that you check out their skin closely and document everything appropriately. This means checking out wounds, in between folds, bony prominences, etc. To preserve the privacy and dignity of my younger completely oriented patients, I wait to take a peek at their tush until the family is not in the room.

If they have any dressing changes, I wait to look and chart until I'm ready to change it, because it hurts their skin if you're taking tape off multiple times around a sensitive wound. If I'm not ready to change the dressing, I wait to look at the wound. However, use your nursing judgment. If you think it'll be hours before you can change the dressing, go ahead and peel the dressing back to take a look and replace it. You shouldn't go a long period of time without laying eyes on it. You need to make sure signs of infection are not setting in.

If they're morbidly obese or a total care patient, I wait until my CNA bathes them to look at their backside, or until it's time to turn them. There's no need to do that right after shift change and again 45 minutes later when your tech does a bath. Cluster your care and manage your time. I manage my time around my total care patient turns. What I mean by this is I do assessments, meds, dressing changes, etc. at or around the time to turn them. If time permits, I typically help my tech give baths to my patients so I can get a good look at everything on the patient, which also builds rapport with my teammates.

Always, always check their butt/coccyx/folds, etc. If it's a hefty boob situation, I'll throw a dry wash cloth on each side. That'll keep it dry and prevent breakdown. You must be consistent with your turns with total care and morbidly obese patients. If they develop a pressure ulcer because you didn't turn them, it's a REALLY BIG DEAL. So if I've done all my assessments and my CNA is nowhere near getting to that bath, I'll grab them to help me turn the patient and take a good butt peek.

(TIP: I'll use this time to also listen to posterior lung sounds if they're difficult to roll. Knock out your lung + skin assessment + a turn in less than a minute.)

And good Lord, do not forget to look at their heels. If they've been in bed for a while, are total care, morbidly obese, have a poor nutritional status, etc., those heels can break down before you know it. I'll lift those gams when I'm having them dorsi/plantar flex and make sure they're not getting red.

All the while, make sure to note if their skin is dry, flaky, pale, bruised, etc.

Now hurry and chart it before you forget!

Medication Errors

Medication errors happen. Don't think you're the worst nurse ever if it happens to you, but, an error occurred, so it's important to take responsibility for it. Below are some of my practical tips to avoiding this:

1. Don't engage family in conversation when administering meds. I hate silence; it feels awkward to me. But I had to get used to being okay with silence while I'm getting meds together and scanned in the room. That's when you make mistakes – when you're distracted.

2. I always double-check my insulin and any other high-alert meds or partial doses with a coworker.

3. I always have a coworker do math separately from me when calculating partial dose medication. Also, if the computer does the math for me, I still double-check it.

4. Pharmacy can make mistakes too; it happens. That's why there are multiple checks (physician, pharmacist, nurse) before the medication actually gets to the patient. Make sure you're checking your order or what you know the doctor wanted against the actual med that's sent up or what you've pulled from Pyxis.

> *Nurse-ipedia definition: A Pyxis is an automated medication-dispensing machine utilized by many health care facilities.*

5. If you have to give half of a pill or a partial dose of an IV push med, cut/draw it up after you scan it when the prompt comes up to tell you that it is a partial dose (if you use a computer med admin system that does that). Errors occur when you're scanning your meds and a pill needs to be cut in half and you think, "Oh, I'll just scan these other three pills real quick and then cut my pill" and then someone interrupts you innocently, and you forget to cut the pill and they end up getting twice the amount of the medication.

6. I also never go do something else mid-med pass unless it's an emergency. People will try to interrupt you with phone calls, patient needs, etc. Just tell them you're passing meds and you'll get back to them once you're done. This is the priority.

7. If you have an error, immediately admit it and correct it. Don't try to act like it didn't happen or it's not a problem. Be honest, and don't be

afraid to admit your mistake. It's okay to be embarrassed, but don't let that keep you from doing your job appropriately. Let your charge nurse know, let the MD know, write yourself up, and move on.

If you work in a wonderful facility that has electronic medical records and you scan your medications as you give them, they make it pretty difficult to give the wrong meds. You have to scan the patient, scan the med, put in the dose, etc., so you have multiple safety checks. They're fantastic. That should never take the place of your nursing judgment, but they really do cut down significantly on the possibility of errors.

If you do have a med error, that doesn't make you any less awesome of a nurse. It's all in how you handle it, correct it, and prevent it from happening again.

What to Do When You Make a Mistake

First, always make sure the patient is stable.

Let the physician know, if applicable. Whenever you have to call an MD to let them know something happened because you screwed up, the best way to start that conversation is, "Dr. Smith... I screwed up." Immediately admit your error, don't try to make it seem like it was someone else's fault. Own it, admit to it, and move on. When you start a conversation like that, typically they want to fix it and not reprimand you. I've had a few MD's who were known for being not so nice, but when I called to tell them I messed up, they were very graceful and understanding.

Let your one-up know, if necessary. This will depend on your institution's policies. Let your charge nurse know, assistant manager, manager, etc. as appropriate.

Write yourself up, if necessary. I've written myself up for mistakes before. I've done this because maybe there's a reason I messed this up and others have as well. Maybe there needs to be a process change to prevent this from occurring in the future. I've also done this because I believe in holding yourself accountable for the mistakes you've made. We're in the most trusted profession in the country, and if your manager has to pull you aside and meet with you to hold you accountable for something you screwed up, that says very little about you.

And finally, move on. People make mistakes. It is just part of life. What matters is the integrity in which you handle the situation in the moment and how you change the way you practice so that you don't do it again. All anyone can ask is for you to do the best you can with what you have been given. If you try to do that day in and day out, no one can fault you for that.

The Man, the Nurse, and the Dementor Foot

After I mastered calling the right physician confidently, could give a great report, and efficiently assessed my patients, I felt like a nursing rock star. I felt like could handle anything. However, during these days as a young pup of a nurse, I was ever so naïve.

On one of the days I was feeling particularly confident (unjustifiably so), I told was by the charge nurse that I was going to admit a patient from the emergency department. This was a typical occurrence. I sat down to look at his chart on the computer before the emergency department called report.

Apparently, this patient hadn't been heard from in a while so his son went to check on him at home. It had been about two weeks since he had seen him. The man was wheelchair bound, living independently in a pretty grotesque environment.

When his son saw him, he immediately called 911 because he "just didn't look right". EMS pulled this wheelchair bound man out of the mess that was his home. They described it to the emergency department staff like "one of those homes on those hoarding shows."

Essentially, the patient was feeling so tired and weak that he couldn't transfer himself from the wheelchair to the toilet anymore. For whatever reason, he didn't let anyone know, he just started going to the bathroom on himself. I'm not sure how long this lasted, but it couldn't have been more than a few days (I pray). There he sat, in the same spot, in his health hazard of a home, for days.

During their assessment in the emergency department, they found large pressure ulcers on the back of both forearms (from resting his arms on the arm rests of his wheelchair) and his butt.

> **Nurse-ipedia definition:** *a pressure ulcer is breakdown of the skin from extended and unrelieved pressure that if not removed can result in extensive irreparable damage that can even go down to the bone.*

In addition to this, they had trouble finding the pulses in his feet, which didn't look so good. After getting him cleaned up, he came up to our vascular surgery floor because they were concerned they would need to remove some toes, if not the entire foot. He was going to get a full workup and some additional scans and prepare for possible surgery.

The man rolled on the floor with a smile on his face. Before I even introduced myself, I smelled something, something that I had never smelled before, something I will never, ever forget. (If you're a nurse, you're already ahead of me here.)

What was that smell you ask?

Rotting flesh. It was rotting flesh.

Upon his arrival, it immediately permeated his entire room and slowly engulfed the hallway. You could smell him about four doors before actually getting to his. It was, quite literally, breathtaking.

I did my typical shallow nurse breathing, but could only be in the room for, at max, five minutes at a time. He was completely oblivious to it all. While technically neurologically intact, something was off. He was clueless about what was going on, despite the emergency department staff explaining it all multiple times.

He was alert, oriented, appropriate, and very pleasant. I managed the first half of my assessment, but had to duck out into the hallway for some fresh air. I reentered with a refreshed set of lungs.

It was now time for me to check out his feet. I pulled off his socks, not prepared to see what I saw.

His toes were black.

Not charcoal or grey. Black. Black like *Dementors from Harry Potter* black. The smell immediately intensified to a magnitude that I was not at all prepared for. I basically held my breath for 30 seconds at a time, taking two tiny breaths in between.

As I looked more closely at his toes, I thought I saw something moving. Perplexed, I leaned about as close as I could without losing consciousness. And there they were in all of their tiny, flesh-eating glory.

Maggots.

I saw two little maggots in this man's Dementor foot. I had the typical, "I need nurse back-up" response and made up an excuse to immediately exit the room.

After my oxygen saturation returned back to normal and my shock subsided, I ran to the nurse's station to begin recruiting.

I couldn't ask just any nurse. I needed one with the strongest stomach who also knew what the heck to do in a situation as ridiculous as this. And I knew exactly which nurse I needed.

(All of you nurses reading this just thought of that nurse on your unit.)

And without hesitation, she immediately responded with everything we needed to do. I felt so reassured in her nursey confidence.

"We need to call infection control and ask them how to kill and dispose of the maggots. We need to let the attending physician know. And we need to get room spray, gowns, masks, double glove, and whatever infection control tells us. Let's do this."

"Ok, this now sounded like a manageable task," I thought. "We will approach this in a systematic way, take care of the problem, and move on."

I felt like we were in the middle of a close basketball game. We just huddled for a quick time out, agreed on a plan, put our hands in the middle of the circle, said, "GO TEAM!" and walked away confidently like we were about to destroy our tiny flesh-eating opponents.

"Let's do this," I thought, in my best Will Smith *Men in Black* voice. All I needed was some sunglasses and an isolation gown that looked like a suit.

Infection control told me to use hydrogen peroxide to kill them, and use a cotton-tipped applicator saturated in it to wiggle them out. A small seal-able plastic container and a red biohazard bag would be their grave that would carry them to the incinerator located in the depths of the hospital.

I paged the physician to let him know about our stomach-churning situation. Expecting him to have some elaborate orders in addition to being shocked beyond belief, I was disappointed in his response. As I frantically explained what I thought was a "stop everything you're doing, especially if you're eating, and listen to this" situation, he merely replied with "gross" and quickly hung up.

My fellow nurse offered a few helpful hints on how to deal with the smell because we were going to be in there until the job was done. Keep in mind; the smell of rotting flesh is very powerful. You need to prepare appropriately if you're going to be exposed to it for an extended period of time.

We gowned up and double gloved. She dabbed the inside of our face-masks with mouthwash to combat the smell. She grabbed room deodorizer, which would only dig a small hole in this mountain of a problem, but was worth the momentary relief it provided. She also soaked a small, 2x2 gauze with mouthwash and pinned it to our gowns to provide a continual flow of scent up to our nostrils, hopefully blocking any stinky air attempting to penetrate our masks.

Her smell prevention plan worked beautifully. We beat the insurmountable odds, withstood the odor, and removed a total of eight maggots from this man's foot, all while maintaining a calm and collected demeanor.

As I was coaxing the last maggot out from in between his first and second toes, I realized that not once during this entire endeavor did I tell him what was going on down there. For all he knew, we were giving him a pedicure! He just sat there, smiling and looking around at his new surroundings.

I looked up to him as he was just sitting there, looking out the window. "Sir," I said. "We just removed eight maggots from your foot."

He furrowed his eyebrows with a confused look and then relaxed his face to a resting smile. "Well," he grinned. "Didn't know I was feedin' a farm down there!"

And that, ladies and gentlemen, was my very first *Nurse Eye Roll Moment*.

CHAPTER 4

Nursey Time Management

You may have heard of the term "time management" before. It is a very essential skill to master as a nurse. You are responsible for doing and charting a lot of things within a 12-hour shift. Because of this, you have to know how to appropriately manage your time to get it all done. If you don't, you'll never clock out. You'll just live at the hospital, and before you know it, you'll be a patient.

In any given shift, you are responsible for completing a certain amount of tasks for each patient in addition to monitoring them and notifying the physician if they start to decline or change. These tasks include, but are definitely not limited to: routinely assessing each patient, administering all medications, changing dressings, educating and discussing with them their plan of care, admissions, discharges, transfers, updating family members/loved ones, participating in rounding with the physicians and other members of the interdisciplinary team, and so forth. You also must document each and every single thing you do because if something isn't documented, it wasn't done.

As you noticed, that is a lot of stuff! You must approach each shift with a plan of attack. You need to know what to do first (or how to prioritize), and how to quickly think on your feet as things change (re-prioritizing!). There is barely enough time in your 12-hour shift to complete everything for each and every person you are responsible for. Therefore, you need to manage the allotted time to ensure your tasks are completed. You also need to ensure that while you're focused on completing tasks, you don't get so wrapped up in your task list that you care about completing that more than you care about doing what's best for the patient. It is easier to slip into that mentality than you may think.

Quick reminder: nursing care is a continual process. I know we would all like to give and receive our patients with all tasks completed and in the best shape possible. However, that's not realistic. Sometimes it happens, but deterioration, admissions, and codes love to happen around shift change. If you feel the previous nurse left you with too much to do, address it before they leave and don't complain to the entire nurse's station about how lazy they are. Deal with it and squash it.

However, if you just have a busy patient with a lot going on, please don't blame the previous nurse. It is not their fault. It's just one of the less awesome aspects of our job. Just like *floating*. It does you no good to be upset with the person in charge who informs you that it's your turn to float.

> **Nurse-ipedia definition:** *floating occurs when your unit is fully staffed, but another unit is short staffed. Therefore, you float to the other unit to help out.*

Again, it's not their fault, it's just part of our job. Please do not let these not so awesome things get to you and make you grouchy. Many people deal with these situations with grace and joy every single day, and these people are ultimately happier, and because of that, people want to be around them. They don't want you to be around you if you complain about a normal part of the job you signed up for. If you act like that, you're one of the nurses everyone else dreads working with. Don't be a cancer to the team.

Time Management on the Floor

I really learned time management well when I worked on an acute-care nursing step-down with cardiac, vascular, and stroke patients. I typically had four to five patients on day shift and five to six on night shift. Report was 30 minutes, and ended at 0730 and 1930. On days, I'd be wrapping up charting at 1030, and on nights, 2300 (given that I didn't get an admission or someone decompensated during that time). First, I'll to cover some general time management tips, and then I'll go into a general timeline.

Nurse Eye Roll's Floor Nursing Points of Enlightenment

1. *Write quickly for report and try not to interrupt with questions.* The faster you get through report, the sooner you can start your day. After the nurse is done giving their report, ask your clarifying questions.

2. *If family members call for an update during or shortly thereafter shift change, tell them (or the person who answered the phone) that you will call them back once you have assessed them and introduced yourself.* That kind of non-emergent stuff can wait until you see what kind of shape all of your patients are in. You'll also be able to give them a better update as well.

3. *Start with your easiest patient first, then progress to your more time consuming patients, seeing the most time consuming patient last.* You would rather be late on one person's medications than be late on four to five patients' medications. If you've charted a little bit as you go along, you'll also be able to spend more time with your most time

consuming patient because you won't have to worry about administering more medications.

4. *Pay attention to time sensitive medications when you're deciding which order to see your patients in.* Insulin is a major one, especially if you work day shift and their breakfast tray arrives right after shift change.

5. *If able, chart in the patient's room right after you complete your assessment.* If you can't chart your entire assessment, chart only the things that are different or abnormal, and go back later to fill in the stuff that is normal or the same for most patients when you have time. You'd be surprised how quickly you forget information.

6. *Do not wait until you've seen everyone and attempt to sit down to chart everything at once.* Rarely will you go 30 minutes uninterrupted to chart, so you might as well do it in the room where people are less likely to bother you. Charting in the nurse's station is a no go; there will be constant interruptions.

7. *Save your non-emergent/urgent questions for when the doctor rounds.* Things that may have seemed like an emergency in nursing school aren't so much of an emergency in the real world. You don't need to drop everything and page the doctor at 0740 because you have a question about an order. If it's something that can wait for the doctor to round, just hang on until they come by the unit.

8. *Don't go do something else in the middle of passing medications.* Someone may say, "Hey can you help me get Mr. Smith on the bedpan real quick?" while you're scanning your meds. Don't do it! This is when medication errors occur! Let them know you're in the middle of passing meds to this patient and once you're done, you'll help them.

9. *Knock out your meds, assessment, and charting all at once.* I know it's not always possible, but this is the most efficient way to completing care. I like to walk into the room, put my meds down and go assess my patient. Then, I'll scan all of my medications, and while the patient is taking them, I'll chart my assessment. The information is fresh, you have some time to build rapport with the patient and family, and you don't have to worry about finding time later to document.

Floor Nursing Timeline

Efficiency, prioritizing and re-prioritizing are key here to time management.

Let's say I'm walking around, getting report on my five patients. I tell them all who I am, that I'll be back with meds and to do my assessment, and if there's anything going on today (for example, going to get an MRI, x-ray, etc.).

This lets them know *I'll be back so don't ask me for anything right now* in a polite, *I still care about you but have a lot to do* way. When you over-communicate with your patients and families, that cuts down on call lights asking to see their nurse when they just need to ask you a question. Maximize that time at the bedside with thorough communication.

I make a quick exit because I have a lot of care to coordinate for the five patients I currently have in addition to the additional two I'll probably receive this afternoon.

Then I run back to the nurse's station (hopefully before anyone needs anything) and see who has 0730 or 0800 meds or breakfast insulin and say what's up to my CNA's.

"HEY CNA's – how are you today? Gah, that Starbucks looks delicious. The guy in room 73 uses the urinal but needs help or else we'll have 10 total bed

changes on our hands, 82 is a high fall risk that almost fell last night, and 83 will be discharged really early today. Let me know when you're giving baths and I'll try to help. GO TEAM!"

After report, I can collect my thoughts about each patient and decide which order I would like to see each of them. Those patients with insulin and early meds get assessed first. However, if I found out in report that a patient or loved one is extremely chatty, I save them for last so I'm not late on any medications.

Additionally, it's always important to see who has blood sugar checks when deciding which patient to see first. Generally speaking, that should be one of your medication priorities. I always got excited when I didn't have a patient who needed insulin (cough-never-cough-cough). Insulin is time sensitive and you'll be surprised how many patients forget to tell you they've eaten 45 minutes ago, despite being a diabetic for 12 years. You really need to stay on top of those blood sugars by asking your CNA's if they've been completed and keeping an eye on when trays arrive.

Once my plan of attack has been decided, I head for the first room, supplies in hand. As I said before, I go in and introduce myself first. Then I assess the patient from head to toe. I then scan and administer my medications. While they're taking their meds, I sit down at the bedside computer and chart the assessment I just completed. If I don't have time to chart the entire assessment, I just chart the abnormal things (for example, if I needed a Doppler to assess their pedal pulses, if they had expiratory wheezes, or if they were confused) and go back and chart the normal things later when time is no longer a constraint.

Some nurses chart all of their assessments after they've seen all of their patients. I tried that, but I mixed things up and forgot some information, which forced me to go back and reassess. I would lose the time I saved by not charting in real time. It's also difficult to find 30-45 minutes to sit down and chart absolutely everything for 5-7 patients without interruptions. I found this to be inefficient.

Charting in the room in the beginning is important because you're not going to be able to chart a full assessment in two minutes like you will in one to two months from now. And this is also helpful when you forget to ask them something—you don't have to get up and walk to their room. You can just ask them really quick and move on. Also, don't feel like you're annoying your patient by charting in there. This is hospital life in 2014 – computers in the rooms and nurses doing their charting at the bedside. You're in charge. You're the nurse. Get your charting done.

Delegation is also important at this busy time. If you're giving meds/assessing and they want to do something that will take more than three to seven minutes, get the tech to do it when you're done. It sounds mean, but you honestly do not have time. You should spend approximately 15 minutes with each patient between charting and meds. If you spend 20-25 minutes with each, you'll be late on your meds. I used to do this because I felt bad. I was in with everyone for 30-45 minutes each, doing all their morning care. It does not work! Delegate in a non-jerky, all-business kind of way.

This timeline, without interruptions, should get you done with all charting/meds by 1000-1015.

Delegation

Delegation is an essential part of nursing. Truly, if you are carrying a full patient load, you do not have the time to provide total care to all of your patients. Tasks must be delegated to your CNA's (if you have them!) consistently and appropriately throughout your shift.

The NCLEX talked a lot about which tasks to delegate, but it didn't necessarily tell you *how* to delegate. Furthermore, it didn't go into delegating to experienced CNA's when you're a brand new nurse that's new to the culture on the unit. Honestly, it can be more intimidating than when you delegate to your new fellow nurses.

Like I said before, I would get very far behind because I was too intimidated to delegate to the CNA checking their email. I honestly have to just get over myself, delegate the task, and follow up if it wasn't completed.

Nursing is a little different than many other fields. You go through a lot with your coworkers, and because of that, you tend to get really close. This closeness is amazing and supportive, however sometimes it can be enabling. At the end of the day we're all here to take care of the patients, friendships or no friendships. We all need to hold each other accountable and complete the jobs in which we are paid to do.

To avoid the feeling of inconveniencing a friend when delegating, I recommend delegating in a matter-of-fact, all-business sort of way with a professional tone, rather than a "can you do me a favor" type of tone. When you present a task as a favor, you present it as something in which they have the option not to complete.

Please don't misunderstand me here. I understand that CNA's also have a lot of tasks to complete, and sometimes they do have to tell the nurse, "I'm sorry, I am absolutely swamped right now and really behind. Is there anyone else available?" I get that. I was a CNA. However, that is very different from delegating a task to someone sitting in the nurse's station Snapchatting and checking Facebook. In that instance, if something is appropriately delegated, it must be completed promptly.

Whether you're younger than your CNA's, close in age, or friends, you're the nurse. It is ultimately your responsibility to insure the tasks are completed for your patient. So when you're at work, even if you're friends, there needs to be a certain level of professionalism maintained so that they know when you're delegating, it is not an option.

I know I sound kind of mean, but this is the reality of how the CNA and nurse need to work together. There is absolutely no point to having CNA's if we're not delegating appropriately. Inappropriate delegation means that you're not being efficient.

Being a CNA is tough work. I've been there. I worked as one during nursing school, did a nursing internship, and went through nursing school. However, because the job isn't the easiest does not justify not delegating appropriately. When you delegate, it's nothing personal. It's not that you're trying to make someone's day tougher; it's just the job in which they signed up for. So if you're swamped and your patient just urinated all over their bed, and your CNA is hanging out at the nurse's station, you must delegate the task to them. It can feel like you're dumping on them, but honestly you're not. Yes, you are perfectly capable of addressing that situation. However, your time would be utilized much better to do those things that only you, as the patient's nurse, can do.

Sometimes it's hard for CNA's that are not in nursing school to truly understand the gravity of the amount of tasks you're responsible for completing in one shift. I always felt like, "they're complaining about charting hourly rounds and I'm constantly charting every single thing I do! All medications, all orders, all education, care plans, changes in status, and, I have to talk to 10 different doctors, answer 40 phone calls, have conversations with families, and still complete the tasks themselves as well! If only they understood!"

Well, the reality is that some CNA's understand and some don't. When I first started as a nurse, I worked with a great bunch of CNA's. On one of my first days, I tried to stay and help clean a patient up despite the fact that I was on the verge of tears because I had so much to do I didn't even know what to do next. I started to help and the CNA said, "Kati, you have a million other things to do that I can't help you with. I've got this. Go." If I hadn't of just met her, I would have hugged her and bought her a friendship bracelet. (High-five Joanna, you're so awesome to me!)

There is an economical side of this as well. If you aren't delegating appropriately and you're always clocking out late, and your CNA's that work with you always get out super early (because you never had them do anything all day!), it costs more money. It costs more money to pay you overtime than it does to pay them their normal wages. It will also stress you out and you'll be exhausted.

Conversely, if your CNA is drowning and you're caught up, please don't spend 15 minutes tracking them down to delegate another task to them that you're completely capable of taking care of independently. To be blunt, that is just really crappy to do. Being a nurse does not mean you're above giving a bed bath, cleaning a poopy patient, walking a patient down the hall, or taking someone to the bathroom. It's a team effort, so if you exclusively separate your responsibilities from the rest of your team, you alienate yourself. If you never offer support to others, then when you are in need it will be nowhere to be found.

So when I find myself delegating to someone who is not responding, I find it best to do so in a systematic, all-business kind of way.

Side note: if someone is consistently refusing or responding very poorly when they are instructed to complete the minimal job expectations, that needs to be moved up the chain. It is important to hold them accountable for the job in which they are being paid to do. I say this because the first thing your manager will ask when you go to talk to them about it is, "did you talk about this with them directly?" Yes, it'll be uncomfortable to address them, but it's necessary. If this behavior is tolerated consistently, it becomes the expectation that when they show up for work, barely anything gets done and they offer no support. Then the CNAs that do a good job end up being asked to the tasks the lazy one refuses to do, which is .. well, just terrible.

However, we tell people how to treat us. If you delegate to someone and they respond rudely to you, and you allow that, they will only continue because they know you'll take it. Not everyone has a great attitude. It can be very stressful to be completely overwhelmed, only to be disrespected when attempting to lighten the load. As much as you're able, don't tolerate people being rude to you; it is not appropriate. Remember, even though things get relaxed on the nursing unit, it is still a professional environment and people need to be held to professional standards.

Furthermore, delegation doesn't just apply to your relationship with CNAs; it applies to your nursey coworkers as well. If you're caught up and someone else is drowning, go see what you can do for him or her to get caught up. Or if you're drowning, ask someone who is caught up to help you out. There is absolutely no reason one person should be flipping through his or her phone at the desk and someone else is an hour behind.

The entire unit is a team; it's not nurses and CNAs isolated with their respective patients. Help each other out when it's needed. Everyone's day will run smoother if everyone knows that if things start going downhill, everyone has each other's back.

The response, "that's not my patient," should never be spoken by a CNA or a nurse. All patients on the unit are everyone's responsibility. We all watch out for one another. While patients are assigned to specific nurses and CNAs; that does not mean we cannot help patients not assigned to us when it is needed.

So please, delegate gracefully. Hold each other accountable. Help out your teammates. Give great patient care. Take the time to say thank you when someone is doing a great job. Rock through your shift without being overwhelmed because you know your coworkers have got your back, clock out, and go home!

Time Management in Critical Care

Critical care nursing is very different from floor nursing. It is less task management on multiple patients and more in-depth big picture thinking on two patients. The stakes are a bit higher and everything is time sensitive. Your high stress level is not because you have a lot of tasks to complete, it's because people are acutely decompensating and it is your job to immediately address it. It's a very different kind of stress, but stress nonetheless.

You can have patients with subarachnoid hemorrhages who are suddenly developing hydrocephalus, septic patients on four different drips, active GI bleeds profusely bleeding from their rectum, patients with impellas that cannot move a muscle, and very emotional family surrounding everyone all the time. Oh, and the guy next door has basically been coding for the last two hours.

First, I will go over some points of enlightenment, and then I will discuss my ideal timeline

Nurse Eye Roll's Critical Care Points of Enlightenment

(While I've written these for critical care, these points can be applicable to step-down and floor nursing as well)

1. *Have a consistent routine.* If you do this, then you won't miss things. Rarely do things work perfectly, but you need to have a consistent, efficient, and comprehensive routine that you stick to when circumstances allow. Otherwise you could miss something important. Additionally, this can prevent you from getting behind early because time quickly can get away from you.

2. *Stay ahead.* Always have your charting done, even if you think you have nothing pressing going on. Things change quickly and severely in intensive care. You could all of a sudden get a coding admission and be in that room for hours, and if you didn't have your stable patient's assessment charted from two hours ago, you'll never remember it now! So if you're ahead on your meds but aren't caught up on charting, it is NOT time to go grab coffee. Chart everything first and make sure there is absolutely nothing left for you to do before you take a break.

3. *Anticipate and prepare.* Once you're there for a little while, you'll be able to predict how patients respond to certain things. For example, if I have a patient with a history of congestive heart failure who needs four units of fresh frozen plasma, I know we're going to need some Lasix at some point; otherwise, Mr. Smith is going to turn into Mr. Respiratory Distress. Additionally, if we're about to do a bedside tracheostomy placement, I know I'll need to have a bolus primed and ready to go. Typically they become hypotensive with the procedural meds we administer. If you anticipate and prepare, you won't have to frantically grab supplies while your patient is decompensating. Every second counts.

4. *Be meticulous.* Most nurses in intensive care have Type-A personalities and are very meticulous and detailed. If you don't care about the details, you can miss something BIG and it would be your fault. Meticulous nurses save lives because they know everything about their patient. And not only that, they care about the details. Say goodbye to being task-oriented—you are now big-picture oriented and you won't be able to see and interpret the big picture if you don't know the details off the top of your head. Additionally, when things go downhill (because they will, and quickly!) you will immediately know the important stuff for quick problem solving in the midst of chaos.

5. *Figure out what you think about death.* I know this is odd to say, but I highly recommend soul searching to figure out what you personally believe happens after people die. Because you're going to see it. A lot. It can be pretty gut-wrenching, and it can hit close to home. Make sure you have a good emotional support system so when you do have a really sad day, you can go talk to someone you trust and love. Nurses who don't have someone to talk to become angry, sad, jaded, and difficult to be around. Moral distress is the number one cause of caregiver burnout. If you can't process that stuff, it'll get to you eventually. PTSD in critical care nurses is real (and in all nursing units); please take care of your heart and soul.

6. *Develop rapport with your physicians.* Like I said before, things change very quickly in critical care. However, sometimes you just get a feeling about something, and you need doctors that will listen to you, even when you don't have something concrete to tell them. Take the time to get to know them and develop a trusting relationship with them. It will pay off not only for you and the physician, but for your patients as well.

7. *7Don't trust the previous nurse. Verify everything yourself.* "But I got in report that…" is not an excuse. You need to verify your orders yourself. Just because the previous nurse said their blood pressure limits were 180-220 doesn't mean they are unless you physically see it in the chart. Rarely is this intentional or neglectful. Maybe they trusted the previous nurse who actually looked at the order wrong and it's just been passed along and no one verified it. So read the physician's notes, look at CT scans, pull up their labs, look at their MAR, etc.

8. *When you come home, process your day with a loved one for no more than 10 minutes, and then move on.* It's very easy to let your nurse life take over your entire life. Don't let it. Yes, you're a nurse, but that is one aspect of your life. Invest and grow the other areas of your life so that work doesn't take over. It will help in dealing with rough work situations when you find fulfillment and purpose in other things. You will get burnt out if you don't maintain a good work-life balance. And that includes unnecessarily going over situations that happened at work that you cannot change. This will not help you, it will only take from you.

9. *Take care of yourself on your days off.* REST, work out, eat right and spend quality time with people you love and who love you. Be intentional with your time. Our job is hard. It's emotionally and physically draining. It's hard to care for patients if you are not caring for yourself.

Critical Care Timeline

As you can imagine, the way you approach your day in critical care is very different than the way you approach your day on another unit. Here is my general timeline after I get report on my two patients. Typically, one is sicker than the other.

After report, I double-check my orders.

I make sure my monitor matches my ordered parameters (for example, if my order is to keep their systolic blood pressure 120-150, I make sure the monitor is set appropriately). I check if there's anything I have to do (meds, labs, scans, etc.) for 0800.

I print and interpret my telemetry strips. If my patients are on drips, I insure I have a full bag and one on deck. If not, I order one.

I plan to go see my sicker patient first. I get any 0800 meds and supplies, go in and complete my assessment, turn them, give meds, do oral care, and talk to them about the plan for the day. If time allows, I immediately chart my assessment at the bedside.

I check all lines and tubes to ensure everything is in date and where it needs to be. This allows me to mentally organize my day. *"Ok, I need to change my tube feeding bag at 1600 and grab a new bag of fluid and tubing with my 0900 meds.."* I level, zero, and calibrate all lines at this time as well.

Then, I go grab any 0800 and 0900 meds and supplies for my second (less sick) patient. I complete everything listed above with this patient and immediately chart what I've done. I usually end up administering medications last because it's barely 0800 by this time and I have to wait until then to give my 0900 meds. So sometimes I even chart my entire assessment first and then go back to administer meds.

Then I head back into my first patient's room with their 0900 meds. If they are a q2h neuro check (meaning a full neurological assessment needs to be completed and documented every two hours), I then complete it and chart it at this time.

If my second patient is a q2h neuro check, I then complete that and document.

Typically, if no one decompensates or needs to travel, and if no doctors round, I'm caught up by 0930.

It's an ideal timeline. However, it doesn't happen too often like that. Sometimes you come in, and someone is not doing well at all; and so they absorb your time and attention for a while. But it's important to know your "this is what I do every day when time allows" routine.

CHAPTER 5

Shift Life

Shift work is not easy. Twelve-hour shifts are really not easy; especially 12-hour shifts that are realistically 13-14 hour shifts. You have to approach them with intention or they will take over your life. Instead of being in the driver's seat, you will find yourself falling asleep in the back or getting angry that it's not taking you where you thought you were going.

A 12-hour shift is a long time. Typically 0700-1900 means you have to get there early and leave late. Add in time to commute and getting ready, you're looking at a minimum of a 16-hour day. If you live over 30 minutes from work, you're looking at getting less than an hour or so to eat dinner, de-stress, and shower before you need to be asleep to get less than 8 hours of sleep for the next shift.

As you can imagine, your time on these days is precious. You have to plan accordingly so that you can maximize your time at home to recharge for the next shift.

I make sure to do as much as possible on my days off. I do all of my laundry, grocery shopping, cleaning, etc., so that the only things I need to worry about on the days that I work are working, eating, showering, and sleeping. (Keep in mind, I do not have kids!)

I'm a bit of a planner, and I like to have the least amount of things to do on my days on as possible. I set out my scrubs and pack my lunch the night before. I try to make sure I have a yummy and healthy lunch to look forward to. Sometimes when your shift is really stressful, a delicious lunch that you don't have to go to the cafeteria for can be your saving grace.

As far as exercise is concerned, I work three days a week, exercise three days a week, and take one day off completely to rest. I always make sure I make time to exercise and do things that are non-nurse related.

I played basketball in college before nursing took over my life, so I've grown up lifting weights. My husband is a former athlete as well. We like to make time to work out together and hold each other accountable. It's really helpful to have a workout buddy.

Noms / Eating

Twelve-hour non-stop shifts can be pretty rough on your body. You have to make sure you're eating well to insure you continue to be healthy and don't gain weight.

Things can be so busy that you either forget to eat, or don't have time to eat anything. You can go from the time you leave for work (0530-0600ish) and not even have a sip of water until 1300 if you're not thinking about it!

Typical Nursey Pitfalls

After being immersed in nursing unit culture for a few years, I figured out some of the easiest ways for me to set myself up for failure in the nutrition department. Below are some common things that I've noticed over the years that have been a struggle for me.

1. *Eating the donuts, cake, cupcakes, cookies, chocolates, Edible Arrangements, etc. that someone left in the breakroom.*

    A very thankful family or patient brings in donuts for the staff as a treat. Or it's someone's birthday. Or we outperformed on something. Before you know it, there's a box full of sugary treats in the break room. Since it's been six hours since you've eaten anything, and you only have two minutes to consume something and get your blood sugar out of the 50's... you might as well make it count, right!? I've been there. I've done that. I'm not going to say you can't even have anything like that or lie to you and tell you I didn't do that last week. BUT, be aware of what you're consuming. One donut quickly turns to two. If you're going to allow yourself a delicious donut, try to consider that when you make other meal and snack choices throughout the day. And, if you eat donuts/sugary treats every time you work, you'll start to crave it with each shift. Before you know it, it'll be hard to go a shift without one. Limit your intake; discipline your mind (as Snape would say) when you see those donuts magically appear in the break room!

2. *Ordering out at work.*

    So one of your coworkers decides they're going to order out and starts making their rounds to see who wants to order something. I don't know about you, but when I spend money on delicious food, I like to ensure I have the time to enjoy it while it is warm. Now, just because you've ordered out doesn't mean you get to go eat as soon as it arrives and get your entire break. Rarely do the stars align to allow such a glorious lunch. My advice is to just bring your own food and stick to it. You'll spend less money. You'll eat healthier. You'll be able to enjoy your entire break (hopefully). And you won't have to stress about getting to eat lunch whenever the food arrives. And then when you actually spend the money to eat out, you'll be able to enjoy it and it'll be more of a treat/enjoyable experience for you. Am I telling you that I've never eaten out at work or telling you never to do so? No! I would save the times for ordering out for someone's last day or birthday. That way I could be part of the team without constantly spending money, eating whatever sounded good and not what was good for me.

3. *Not preparing.*

Unless extenuating circumstances present themselves, I always bring my lunch. I go grocery shopping and plan my lunches to ensure they're something I'll enjoy and look forward to. Part of my "night before work" routine is packing my lunch. This way if I wake up late, I won't forgo making my lunch because I don't have time. Once again, be intentional and proactive about your time! However, we all know there are those shifts that are really rough. You get home a few hours late just to be back again in the morning. After one of those shifts, the last thing I want to do is make my lunch. To prepare for these circumstances, I allot myself $20/month to spend on whatever I want at work. This keeps me from overspending and from feeling like I can't ever get anything at work.

4. *Not snacking consistently during the shift.*

My lunch consists of my main meal, a midmorning snack and a late afternoon snack. I don't always get time to snack, but I want to make sure I have something. I'm always starving around 1000 and 1630. If I don't have something quick to eat, I'll make bad decisions out of hunger.

Keep in mind, even if you don't gain weight from eating unhealthy food, your body still has to process all of the artificial ingredients you're consuming and be deprived of the nutrients you are not consuming. A slender figure and the ability to eat whatever you want without gaining weight does not mean you're healthy.

Living the Noc Life

Working night shift can be tough on your body, especially when you're doing it for the first time while working a brand new and scary job! In addition to figuring out how to eat properly, I had to figure out how to maximize my time off so that I was not a zombie when I woke up. It took my body a while to adjust. Here are some hints to getting good, continuous sleep during the day while Living the Noc Life.

1. *Buy good blackout curtains.*
   These will be a worthwhile investment. You need to sleep in a quiet and dark environment during the day, and these will be so important. I got some great ones from Target that weren't too expensive. Keep in mind that, short of sleeping in a room with no windows, there's no way to completely block out the light. Don't be mad when you put them up and you can see some light. It's impossible unless you duct tape them to your wall.

2. *Get a loud fan or something with white noise to drown out the sounds of the day.*
   Someone will start to mow their lawn, someone will come home and accidentally slam the front door, or your dogs will bark. Try to drown out sounds because it will not be silent in the middle of the day unless you live alone with no other home or building for miles.

3. *Turn off your ringer on your cellphone and just have an alarm on.*
   People will forget what days you work and that you sleep during the day. The last thing you want is to have your precious sleep interrupted

because some friend wanted to text you yet another picture of their child that looks exactly like the last picture they texted you.

4. *Have a routine with your spouse or roommate(s).*

   My husband intermittently works nights as well, and we have a routine when one is sleeping during the day. I keep the shades drawn so the dogs don't start barking. I shower in the guest bathroom after my workout so he doesn't wake up. I ask him before he goes to sleep what time we need to eat dinner. I just make sure to lay low that day and be respectful of his sleep. He does the same for me when I work nights. This allows us to maximize our sleep and therefore decrease the grumpies.

5. *Talk to your doctor.*

   This is important if you're starting nights for the first time and you take multiple medications. You may need to change the time that you take them (under your doctor's direction). If you have trouble sleeping during the day and need something to help you sleep, you can talk to him or her about this as well.

6. *Have some snacks that you can quickly eat when you wake up starving at 1200.*

   It never failed. I would always wake up around 1200 ravenous every single day that I slept. I just wanted to quickly eat something and head back to bed. If I didn't have anything healthy to quickly eat, I'd eat junk.

"Flipping" For Night Shift

The hardest part about working nights (for me) was coordinating my sleep schedule so that I was functional on my days off. I've talked to quite a few noc shift nurses and there seem to be three main ways to do this. Some people "flip" every day (being awake during the day, asleep at night), some do if they have more than one day off, and some never flip (always awake at night and asleep during the day). It all depends on what you want to do and your other commitments.

Let's say I'm working Monday, Tuesday, and Friday of this week. To prepare to be up all night, I stay up until at least 0200 on Sunday. I'd go to sleep then until about 0900. I'd get some stuff done around the house (nothing crazy). Then I would take a two-hour afternoon nap, after which, I would get up, get ready, and go to work.

I'm not a heavy coffee drinker—if I have more than two cups, I'm tachycardic and hypertensive. So I space them out. One cup on my way to work; one cup at 0200. If it's past 0300, I stay away from the coffee so I can get to bed after I get home.

Monday-Tuesday is easy because I just go to bed as soon as I get home and wake up around 1700 to eat my dinner and head to work.

When I get off work Wednesday morning, I go to bed immediately when I get home. I set an alarm for 1200 or 1300. I may be exhausted, but I force myself up and drink some coffee. Then, I go to bed at a normal time that night and consider myself "flipped." I sleep that entire night, usually getting up pretty early the next morning. I then prepare for my Friday shift like I did for my Sunday shift.

If I only have one day off in between workdays I don't flip. It's just too much effort for my sleepy head to go through. I do know some people that do, and it works for them, but it was too much for me.

Don't drink the highly caffeinated sodas... or any sodas!

Soda/pop/whatever you want to call it, diet or not, is terrible for you. I forced myself to start drinking coffee. Why am I hating on sugar, you ask? I want to encourage you, as a nurse, to look at the latest research regarding health and nutrition. There are a lot of articles and research studies out there showing that fat is not what is killing us, sugar and hydrogenated oils are. My favorite nutrition blog is called Authority Nutrition (authoritynutrition.com) and it is written with an evidence-based approach to all topics. Every single post references multiple research studies (with links!).

I encourage you to go to that site, check it out, and search for "sugar," "diet soda," and "heart disease" in the search bar on the right hand navigation and read the top three to four posts about them. That's why I <u>never</u> drink diet soda and that's why if I drink soda (or sweet tea, Gatorade, juice, lemonade), it's as a dessert/treat and not a normal part of a meal.

At the beginning of my nursing career, while working nights, I would drink a caffeinated soda halfway through the night to keep awake. I started gaining weight. So I basically forced myself to start drinking coffee because of the dramatic difference in sugar content. One packet of sugar is approximately 3 gms and I like two packets in my coffee with some creamer. At most I am consuming 6 gms of sugar, rather than the 30-40 gms in a regular soda or all of the chemicals/artificial sweeteners in a diet soda. It perks me up, tastes delicious, and is cheaper and healthier.

This is Un-RULY!

I know what you're thinking—this is a lot of rules to live by. However, I did not get to this point over night. I'm telling you what I've find-tuned my routine to after four years of screwing it up. I had to mess up a bunch to figure out that this is what works for me.

It does sound like a lot to think about every single day, but I found that if I had a routine and disciplined myself, I just felt better and had better control over my life. I didn't just order food based on what I was craving, or grab a pop because I wanted to. I just ate what I brought and didn't give myself the option to eat something else. I made sure to have all of my stuff together and organized so I wouldn't have to take a 30-minute trip to the grocery store after a horrendous 14-hour shift. I didn't compromise my sleep schedule for anything unless it was very urgent or an emergency.

Working these long 12-hour shifts can get a little depressing, especially if it means you miss out on some stuff in the rest of your life because of it. The more active role I had in my little every day decisions made such a difference.

I knew nurses who just ate and drank whatever they felt like all through-out their shifts and gained weight over the years. That behavior is hard to break and correct after years of passively doing whatever you want. Starting out with having an active role and control over your eating, sleep-ing, and living choices, and not giving yourself the option to do poorly will hopefully make things easier for you. You can worry about learning how to be a great nurse, not about losing weight, trying to eat better, or just trying to have joy. Being a new nurse is stressful enough; we don't need anything else to worry about!

Does this mean I was crazy strict all the time and hated my life because of the rules? No. It could get a little daunting, but the overall result and con-trol over myself was better than that freedom of eating any and everything. (Although, it becomes harder to control over time so it isn't a freedom anymore.) I'll have a slice of cake during nurse's week, or have a cookie or two if someone brings them, and definitely a donut (I *love* good donuts). But I don't order pizza one night, Chinese the next, McDonald's the next, and have cookies/cakes/soda for regular every day snacks.

Adequate and challenging exercise is also an essential piece of the puzzle. Again, I never work out on the days I also worked on the floor; it's just too much in one day and would compromise my sleep. I'm not a crazy workout-all-the-time person, running marathons, taking pictures of my abs in the mirror and posting them on Instagram, and biking 20+ miles and whatnot. I go to the gym and lift for 30-45 minutes and/or do some sort of cardio/plyometrics. I don't like to work out for more than an hour, because that sounds terrible. I wish I liked working out more, but I do it out of necessity not because it's something I enjoy. It also helps after a terrible shift. I take my frustration out on the work out, feel better, and move on.

Work life balance is important no matter the profession. I believe that when working nights or 12-hour shifts, you do have to take a more active role in maintaining a healthy work life balance because it's so easy to just stop trying. For some people, this comes more naturally. Not me, though. I had to work at it, figure it out over time, hold myself accountable, and let my husband in on everything. It's important to make sure your spouse knows what lifestyle habits you need to have to maintain a healthy work/life balance. Clue your spouse in on what you need/want from him or her and approach these things as team so that you're all on the same page.

Don't think those first few weeks on night shift I didn't flip out on him for being so incredibly loud during the day. He actually wasn't. I was being dramatic and emotional from the stress of work, lack of sleep, and most importantly, a lack of communication about my expectations of how he was to support me while going through this transition. Now I know what I need from him when I work nights. I know what he needs from me. We've communicated about our expectations (for example you have dinner ready when I get up and I'll make time to do the dishes before I leave). Doing so removes a huge burden of stress and festering frustration from us both, and in turn, we are happier and more satisfied with our jobs and marriage.

Communicate, plan, eat right, exercise, take time off, and hold yourself accountable for your decisions every day. Be intentional with how you go about your day and your life. This will give you control and you will find it so much easier to make the right decisions during stressful and compromising situations.

CHAPTER 6

The Tough Ones

===

While most of the time your patients are compliant and want to do what they can to get out of the hospital, not all of them are as agreeable. I was grossly unprepared to deal with mean, demeaning patients. I was also grossly unprepared to deal with difficult patients who, because of their medical conditions, were uncooperative.

Mean and demeaning patients are where my Nurse Face comes out. My "it just got serious" face. If you've been a nurse for more than 12 minutes, you know that some people are, well, jerks. Just like life outside of the hospital environment, some are just not nice people.

Remember, there are many reasons why patients can be difficult. They could have just received a life altering diagnosis. They could be painfully frustrated by the lack of support from their family. They could normally use alcohol or smoking to deal with stress at home, but right now they can't use their normal coping mechanism. They could have underlying mental health issues that are impairing their judgment or perception of reality. There are a lot of very real and understandable reasons that could impede a nurse's ability to provide care to certain patients.

An important thing to fully understand is which battles are worth fighting.

For example, if my super irritated patient detoxing from alcohol is flipping out about me wanting him to take medications, I'm not going to spend 20 minutes convincing him to take his scheduled stool softener. The stool softener is not a priority anymore. His blood pressure medications and *Ativan* are.

> *Nurse-ipedia definition: Ativan is typically given to patients withdrawing from alcohol to combat the symptoms, which can include seizures, delirium tremens (DT's), and especially agitation.*

I'm going to crush those and throw it in some applesauce and try to get him to take that one bite for me. And if I think it's going to be a problem, I'll call my buds in security to stand right next to me to make sure he takes them. And when the doctor rounds, I'll FYI him or her.

And please, do not get into a power struggle for the benefit for your ego. Nurses who get the most bent out of shape by these patients usually have quite a bit of an ego/control thing and flip out when the patient doesn't do as they're told. Getting mad about this is worthless; it'll just stress you out more and make it more difficult to care for them and your other patients.

There are different ways patients can make caring for them difficult. Here are a few different situations and how I typically deal with them.

Grouchy/grumpy/mad about doing anything: Befriend them, joke with them, figure out something they like or care about and bring it up a few times. Be on their side. And then when you need them to do something, present the task as a favor.

Belligerent/combative: You must have a strong and confident presence with these patients. Always immediately stop them if they curse at you and calmly inform them that they will not speak to you in that manner. I never hesitate to call security if someone is combative and difficult to physically control. Know how to tie restraints, how to push Haldol, and the number for security. You must insure you have the appropriate orders for both chemical and physical restraints, if they are needed. Unfortunately, both are necessary sometimes. Once you deal with a few of these situations, you'll know what to do and you'll become more confident each time.

As far as safety is concerned, I've never felt unsafe. Security gets to my unit quickly, I can tie a restraint faster than I can open the package that the restraints come in, and can draw Haldol up even faster.

Demeaning: The first thing to remember about patients who are demeaning is that it might not be about you. They could be mad about something else, be it their disease process or something else going on in their life. When someone speaks to me in a demeaning manner, I reply in a very matter-of-fact tone and say something like, "I am here to care for you today, however it is not appropriate to speak to me in that manner." Most of the time, that defuses the tension and they feel bad for taking their anger out on their nurse and apologize. If I can try to break down the mean wall and ask them about their lives, that usually softens their demeanor. However, not everyone responds like that and when that happens, I keep my interactions short and intentional. I'll talk more in-depth about this in a little while.

Way too talkative/avoiding doing things: Engage in conversation with them, but know when to stop conversation and have them refocus on the task at hand. I always blame the doctors with these patients and say something like: "The doctor insists you get out of bed three times today, no excuses. Let's get the first one out of the way now." (Thanks, docs!) Again, engage in conversation but frequently redirect conversation to the task at hand.

In addition to patients being difficult to care for, occasionally we have to deal with families and loved ones that are as well.

Generally speaking, most loved ones and families care deeply for the patient and want only the best for them. However, they're stressed to the max, feel very helpless, and are way out of their comfort zone. It's completely understandable that they aren't acting as they normally would.

Please don't misunderstand me when I use the word difficult. I mean that with the utmost respect. I use the word difficult because I honestly don't have a better word. Sometimes their concern for the patient can interfere with providing care.

When you hear in report that the family is difficult, it can mean many different things. It can mean they question absolutely every single thing you do, which makes doing anything at all very time consuming and labor intensive. It can mean they act like you don't know what you're doing, passively demeaning you all day long. It can mean they stare at the monitor and react every time there's even a normal fluctuation in vital signs and don't believe you when you reassure them. It can mean they act as if their loved one is the most important person in the entire unit and make it very difficult to be able to care for your other patients.

It is important to remember that many patients and loved ones are not familiar with the medical system. They don't know when to be concerned therefore everything is concerning. You and the physicians are all speaking a totally different language. They just met you and the physicians, so they don't trust you yet. And they don't live in this medical world every day like you do. Remember to have some extra grace and understanding.

Even if they come off rude, demeaning, frustrated, or passive aggressive, what's usually at the bottom of all of that is *fear*.

First of all, when you hear in report that the family is rough, you need to consciously step up your patience game. You'll need more patience with this today than a normal situation. All of your interactions are going to have to be intentional today. You're going to have to try harder with them than other patients and families because they need it. Everything you do or don't do, they're watching and analyzing. Every time you walk in that room, walk in with confidence, having intentional conversations.

What I mean by intentional is that you have purpose behind everything you say to them. You're not just flippantly chitchatting; you mean business because they are dissecting every word you say.

Below is how I have intentional conversations. It was a little difficult and awkward at first, but now it's like clockwork and I don't think about it anymore.

I always go in the room and introduce myself to my patient first. I tell them my name, that I'll be their nurse all day and I shake their hand. I don't know why, but this simple gesture can mean a lot to someone. It tells them that they are not just another patient to me; they are a person that I am meeting for the first time and am happy to meet them. During my introduction, I speak directly to the patient first. Everything is about them. Family or no family, this person still needs your care and he or she should be the center of everything you do.

During this time, I'm speaking directly to the patient and occasionally look at whomever else is there. When I'm done with that, I ask the patient, "So who is this you've got here with you today?" I always shake their hand as well and introduce myself to them after I've spoken with the patient directly. It sets a professional tone.

If the loved one's already mad, hopefully that defuses their frustration. Maybe they hated the nurse last night and the doctor was short with them yesterday. Maybe no one has really explained to them what's going on and they feel completely out of the loop. There are a million reasons people are rude, overbearing, mean, condescending, etc. However, let them know through your actions and conversation that you are here now. It is a new day and you are a new nurse to the situation, and today we are going to have a fantastic day.

You want them to feel safe and know that you're going to take good care of their loved one. Making your presence and authority known initially tends to make them feel better about leaving their loved one in your care. It reassures them. You want them to trust you. The more they trust you, the more freedom they'll give you to let you care for the patient.

When you have that initial conversation at the beginning of your shift, let them know what the deal is for the day, the goals for the day, when you can loosely predict the doctor will be around, etc. (Use "we" terms, because you're on the patient's team, getting things done for them. It's not the family versus the health care team, we're all on the same team.) Any plans, structure, or routine that you can provide is reassuring.

Predictability is something that reassures even the most scared family members the most; remember that as you're interacting with them. Even if you think you're being redundant, go over the plan again. You are in charge and it enhances your professionalism and authority. It also makes them feel safe and taken care of during a scary and helpless time. Their loved one is in your nursey hands, and that probably scares them because they have no idea who you are and if you know what the heck you're doing.

I try to keep things light as much as possible because patients really enjoy that. Typically, they're in the hospital for something sad/serious/scary, so if you can make them laugh or talk about something not illness related, they light up. If their family member sees them smile, that means so much more to them than getting their meds right on time.

Have you noticed that families are typically more stressed than the patients themselves? I get it; I would much rather be sick myself than see my husband in a hospital bed. I'm nauseated just thinking about it. However, that doesn't excuse inappropriate behavior.

So I give families a little room to push my buttons, but just a little. Sometimes in the heat of frustration or sadness, they can come off short or rude. Again, I understand. I try to have as much grace as possible in these situations, but sometimes you have to draw the line. Using a reassuring voice, I let them vent their frustrations and tell them I understand. Rarely do they say anything about the care I personally am providing. If it starts to get personal, I refocus the conversation on the patient. I get as firm as I need to and stand up for myself, when appropriate.

"I understand that it was really frustrating to hear the doctor say what she said. I know you had a lot of hope that he would walk out of here and she just told you he wouldn't. Keep in mind that we're all on the same team here. We're here to support you both through this. I'm really sorry you're going through this. I'm here for you. We want to be open and honest with you about what's going on, even if it's bad news. We don't want you to be in the dark about the reality of the situation."

Most of the time, the person feels bad right away and stumbles over their words to apologize. Again, it's never about me. It's about the situation and how they deal with whatever is happening to them.

Know that line in your head. Know when things need to get serious and refocus on the patient. That line is different for every nurse. The more aware of that line you are, the more control you have and the less frustrated/mad you'll get when someone starts to cross it and the more confident you will be.

Some nurses get super offended every time someone is kind of rude. They get stressed easily, and it's just not worth it. Just remember people are under immense duress and many don't have a good way to cope with it. Give it very little power in your heart and mind.

Now, these "it just got real" conversations never happen at the end of your shift. They're always two hours in when you have 10 more hours to deal with them. Maintain your professionalism when you have additional interactions throughout the day.

An occasional joke goes a long way. Don't shun that person the rest of the day, it just creates more stress for you and makes caring for the patient more difficult, and is honestly kind of mean and immature on your part if that's how you choose to deal with these situations. Hook your patient up with some ice cream or a warm blanket or something. If they know you're still going to take care of their loved one, they usually chill out eventually.

Dealing with difficult patients and families can become emotionally exhausting if you don't know how to deal with them. Honestly, nursing is already emotionally exhausting that first year or so when you are figuring out how to deal with everything.

I have also noticed a different kind of anxiety exemplified by patients and families when I transitioned into critical care. Things are just scarier in critical care. Scarier means increased anxiety for everyone. There are more beeps, more tubes, lines, drains, machines, and rooms full of sick, sick people.

I'll always remember one family that would have been considered a difficult family but will always be near and dear to my heart.

He was in his 70's and diagnosed with colon cancer a few years prior, received treatment and was in remission for a while. Well, he started to get confused at home and they brought him in and found out the cancer had spread to his brain.

What ended up needing to happen was placement of a ventricular peritoneal shunt due to low-pressure hydrocephalus, however he wasn't stable enough to make it through the surgery. His blood counts were all over the place and neurologically he was in a non-responsive, but awake, vegetative state. The surgery wasn't going to fix his neurological status; it would merely remove the need for the extra-ventricular drainage device called a ventriculostomy.

Every time the monitor beeped, she panicked. Every time he made even the slightest of movements, she rejoiced. It was quite the emotional rollercoaster ride that ended up lasting months.

Rarely could the staff do anything right. Rarely did we get in the room fast enough. Rarely was she pleased with us. It took me a few weeks to realize that she wasn't upset with us; she was upset with the situation. It's almost like coaching a sport. When the team wins, it's their victory. When they lose, it's the coach's fault. I felt like we were his coach and we lost every single game every single day.

After being in the thick of it for weeks, and then months, many of us just couldn't emotionally take it anymore. Out of self-preservation, we'd switch off who cared for him because we were all just so sad for him.

Whenever a physician would come in, she'd focus solely on anything positive he or she might say, no matter how insignificant. It started to take the focus away from the big picture of it all…that he was dying. However, no matter how many physicians came in and told her the same thing, she was still full-speed ahead. The thought of palliative care or hospice was not an option. We ached for him.

Eventually, a few physicians had a family meeting and got through to her that absolutely everything had been done to save her husband, yet he continued to deteriorate and would continue to do so. She finally agreed to transfer to our hospice unit.

Myself, another nurse from my unit, and a physician that was closely involved during their entire stay went and visited them. He was still alive, but finally looked comfortable. It was relieving to see that he was going to be allowed to pass and he didn't have to fight for a futile fate any longer.

I was able to tell the family some things that I couldn't tell them before because I was so frustrated that he was on our unit for so long. I was able to tell her that I'm glad he has a wife that loves him so dearly, and that he clearly loved her deeply. She told me some stories about him and just seemed softer in her interactions. I think it meant a lot to her that we came down to see them that day and offer our condolences.

When he was on our unit, I was frustrated and upset. I hated when I came into work after a few days off and saw him still in our unit. It made me not want to come to work. It made me a little bitter.

But when I went down there to offer my condolences to them, all of that went away. I remembered why I'm a nurse. I remembered why I love my job.

Even the tough patients need us. Even the ones that are mean, cruel, demeaning, or overbearing – they need us, desperately.

CHAPTER 7

The Code Blues

To start out my chapter on code blues, I'd like to share with you my very real first code blue.

My First Code Blue

I was a few weeks out of orientation and working the night shift on my cardiovascular and thoracic surgery step-down unit. Collectively, myself and the other three nurses had all finished our med pass and assessments, and were just sitting down to finish up out documentation. The techs were going around room to room to do vitals. All was well in our nursey world.

One of the telemetry alarms started going off, a usual occurrence on our floor. I looked up from my computer to see the patient's heart rate flashing in red. It was 36.

"Not too bad…I've seen worse," I thought. "She's probably really asleep and normally drops this low. I'll go check on her for my coworker because she's with another patient." I got up and walked to her room across from the nurse's station.

I walked in the dark room, "Ma'am... ma'am..." I said, as I walked closer to her. A coworker was behind me and screamed, "SHE'S NOT BREATHING CALL THE CODE!"

As I rushed to the head of the patient's bed, I thought, "Man, how did she see that? It's so dark in here. I should have noticed that immediately."

Just before the code was called overhead to summon the troops, I heard our emergency red telephone ring at the desk. It was the telemetry monitors that were located on another floor, calling us to tell us the patient had flipped into a deadly heart rhythm.

I frantically searched for the CPR lever that's on all hospital beds and couldn't find it. I gave up and tried to get her head positioned to put the bag valve mask on her face. I didn't know what I was doing. I guessed that was the next best thing to do. The most experienced nurse had her head together. I felt like an idiot. She pulled the CPR lever immediately. She directed the tech to start chest compressions while she slapped the defibrillator pads on the patient. The tech started compressions.

"She needs to push harder, lower, and faster," I thought. "But what do I know? I've never done this before. My experienced nurse didn't say anything so she must be doing okay. I hope."

I heard the code cart coming down the hall. My coworkers rushed the patient's roommate out of the room and down the hall. This wasn't going to be pretty.

The patient had just had open-heart surgery the week before. The large incision down the middle of her chest was still stapled together. The staples were soon soaked with blood from her newly damaged incision.

Respiratory therapy arrived and took over for my fumbling attempts to clear her airway. I took over for CPR. I didn't even put gloves on; I just started compressions. For some reason, I didn't even think about it. All I could think of was minimizing the time between compressions. I did mine harder, lower, and faster. No one said anything.

The ICU nurses, ED nurses, and in-house hospitalist with his residents showed up. They took over. I stepped back and watched, feeling helpless for this poor woman who wasn't half-dead four minutes ago.

They did the typical rounds of IV push meds to get her heart in a normal rhythm. They stuck a breathing tube down her throat. The ICU and ER nurses showed me how to do real chest compressions. The hospitalist made the residents take turns doing chest compressions. They got blood on the sleeves of their freshly pressed white coats.

In the midst of the controlled chaos, the house supervisor asked, "has anyone called the family?"

The family. I forgot about the family.

"Not that we know, we're coding her!" screamed someone in the room. The house supervisor told the charge nurse to call the family and tell them to get here. Now.

I tried to help in any way that I could. I ran to get saline flushes, IV pumps, primed tubing, wrote things down...but somehow felt like I didn't do a thing. I looked at the nurse pulling meds from the code cart seamlessly, the one pushing them in her central line and calling them out with the time so the recorder knew what he was doing, and the one doing compressions so well that I could see it on the monitor.

"How do they know how to do this? ... And how do I not?" I thought.

Thirty-five minutes passed.

Nothing.

"We have been coding her for 35 minutes and have had no response," said the doctor. "We will attempt one more shock and if that doesn't work, we will call it."

"Clear the patient," said the ICU nurse that was at the defibrillator. Everyone stepped back from the patient.

"SHOCKING," she said, as she pushed the blinking orange button.

The shock caused the patient's chest to momentarily jump up off of the bed. We all stared at the monitor in silence.

She flatlined.

"Time of death: 2342," said the doctor as he was taking off his bloody gloves.

Everyone stopped what they were doing, threw away what was in their hands, and immediately left the room. The doctor signed what he needed to and left. The ICU and ER nurses did the same. One of my coworkers printed a telemetry strip of her flatline to put in the chart.

The nurse who was taking care of the patient was crying in the hallway. The family started walking down the hallway towards the nurse's station. We all looked at each other to see who was going to step up and tell them. The doctor was already gone. The daunting responsibility somehow fell on her. Through her tears, the nurse told them she didn't make it.

The patient's brother was stoic as he heard the news.

"She had a cough two days ago and no one did anything about it!" screamed the patient's sister; which just made the nurse cry more.

A few others and myself went into the room to clean her up to make her presentable for the family. We cleaned up all of the blood that oozed out of the foot-long incision on her chest, closed her eyes by holding them down for 30 seconds, and discarded the remnants of the code. The trash-cans were full of empty medication vials, syringes, wrappers, and bloody gloves.

After we gave them the all clear, they filed in and closed the door.

The house supervisor comforted the crying nurse, whose patient just died, and whose family member blamed her. There was literally nothing she could have done differently, and he made sure she knew that. She pulled it together and started charting… she had to call the coroner soon.

The house supervisor went in and asked if they wanted an autopsy, and which funeral home they wanted to go with. Once they said they didn't want an autopsy, we could go in and take out all of her lines and tubes.

I went in and removed her breathing tube, central line, and urinary catheter. I used surgical lube to wiggle her wedding band off of her cold swollen finger to give to her family.

The family went in one more time to see her as they always saw her, without the large breathing tube down her throat and her head cocked as far back as it could go. They left, one by one, with blood-shot eyes and heavy hearts.

I went back in with my tech, put her in a body bag, and put a tag on her foot.

The funeral home was called. They'd be here in an hour to pick her up.

And then I went to go pass my late midnight meds.

Code Blues for Newbies

Cardiac and respiratory arrests are terrifying, whether you've never done it, or only watched it before and now you're in the thick of it! Something that's important to understand with these situations is that unless you're with a highly experienced team, it can get pretty loud and hectic. If someone yells at you during a code, please don't take it personally. That is someone's way, albeit misdirected, of feeling in control in a chaotic situation.

Here are some things for you to do in a code situation when you don't know what to do.

As you may know, *BLS and ACLS* have been updated to where compressions are our number one priority. This must be done before anyone does anything else. Someone needs to be on their chest, cracking their ribs. (Yes, if you feel their ribs break under your hands that means you're doing it right.)

> *Nurse-ipedia definition: BLS (basic life support) nurses can provide CPR and ACLS (advanced cardiac life support) nurses can push meds per the ACLS algorithms without a physician.*

The code cart has a backboard that breaks off and that needs to be placed under the patient. If I hear a code and am running down the hall next to someone else getting the cart, I rip it off and bring it in with me even if compressions aren't indicated yet. Get the backboard under them so compressions can start immediately when necessary.

If someone is taking care of compressions, the next thing to address is the patient's airway. Every single hospital room should have a bag-valve mask connected to oxygen tubing at the head of the bed. Connect it to the oxygen valve on the wall and crank it all the way up. Tilt their head back and seal the mask over their nose and mouth and squeeze the bag to administer breaths. The code cart should have portable suction. If the room doesn't already have suction set up, go ahead and turn that bad boy on. It is used to clear secretions from their airway, which is essential during intubations. Typically, respiratory therapy shows up very quickly and takes over for airway management. It is very helpful to them if you have this set up and started for them to just hop into your place.

In every single code, the defibrillator needs to be attached to the patient. Most code carts are set up to where you unplug the defibrillator from the code cart itself and set it on the bed. The faster this is done, the better. Even if your patient is on telemetry, and had a respiratory arrest and still has a pulse, get the defibrillator on. The pads will indicate where they need to be placed on the patient. Once the pads are on the patient, turn on the defibrillator and position it so that the physician can see their rhythm from where they are standing.

All right, what else do we need? IV access! Make sure the patient has some sort of access. If not, start working on another IV. Prayerfully, they already do and one of your ACLS-certified nurses is pulling meds and drawing them up from the code cart and the other is pushing them.

If you can get chest compressions started, get the bag-valve mask on them, have the defibrillator attached and on the bed, and have IV access, your code team will thank you. It's as if you're a basketball team that only ever runs one play, and the "code blue" being announced overhead is like you're running down the court to get set up. Getting those three things done for them is the perfect set up for them.

Ideally, there are two people for compressions (one actively doing them and one ready to switch), three ACLS RN's (pushing meds, pulling them, and announcing the ACLS algorithm/times), an MD, an RN documenting, one runner, one to two respiratory therapists at the head of bed, and the primary nurse telling the doctor what happened. There shouldn't be more than that in the room. If you were doing something and the code team arrived to take over, immediately exit the room.

Qualities of a Smoothly Run Code

1. It's quiet and calm. No one is shouting. People calmly ask questions and request supplies. No one speaks unless it is pertinent to the care that's being provided.

2. The only interruptions to CPR are during designated pulse checks after two-minute cycles and during shocks (yes, you need to keep doing compressions while the defibrillator is charging).

3. Someone is with the family. It can be easy to forget about them when a code is called; make sure someone is with them. If the family isn't at the bedside, make sure someone is calling them.

4. Everyone moves efficiently. Every second counts.

5. It's documented in real time and orders are entered in real time.

6. The patient's primary nurse tells the physician exactly what's going on with the patient and what led up to the code quickly.

7. Someone is able to look things up quickly and efficiently in the patient's chart (labs, last chest x-ray, recent tests/procedures, etc.)

8. If it's a small room, someone takes out unnecessary items. If everyone that needs to be in the room is, and there's a huge recliner blocking the door, someone move that recliner! Chances are, if the patient survives, the bed will be moved out of the room.

Also, keep in mind that a code run out on the floor runs differently than one in the intensive care unit (ICU) or emergency department (ED). In the ICU or ED, rooms are usually bigger and the nurses, techs, and physicians are more familiar with codes. Patients typically have adequate IV access, they're already hooked up to telemetry, and ventilators and other advanced equipment are really close by. Basically, ICU/ED codes tend to run smoother and are more efficient.

If you have the ability to go to a code in an ICU/ED just to watch, I highly encourage it. It's quite an experience to just sit back and watch. Not to sound weird, but it's almost artistic and beautiful to see this team of people working together to save someone's life. The calm teamwork is amazing to see. The doctor asks for something, it's done immediately. The doctor asks a question, he or she gets an answer. The things that just need to be done (apply defibrillator and turn it on, pop open the intubation kit, get IV access, apply backboard, prime a bolus) are already done or being done. No one has to ask.

Note: ICU and ED CNA's are awesome at CPR. If you want to learn how to do great chest compressions, go watch the CNA's in the ICU and ED. It is exhausting and tiring, but good chest compressions save people's lives. So, shout out to all of you CNA's out there! You make all the difference in the world.

Not everyone in the hospital who dies goes through a code. Many people have predictable (or loosely predictable) deaths. For every code I've gone to, I've sat through ten comfort care conversations. Many times we realize a patient is going to die and need to sit down and talk to the patient and family how about we will proceed.

Comfort Care Conversations

Ideally, the doctor brings this up when they decide nothing else can be done. When you know this is about to happen, you should be in the room. It's tough, but you should. You're there with them all day; your presence should be comforting to them because they see you more than the doctor.

Nurse-ipedia definition: Comfort care means that recovery is no longer our goal of care, and making the patient comfortable as they pass is now the focus.

Sometimes we need to take the palliative care step before hospice or comfort care. Palliative care is different than hospice. You don't have to be dying to receive palliative care. Palliative care basically prevents suffering and relieves pain. You can be a 25-year-old military veteran with an amputation and receive palliative care.

Palliative care is a wonderful thing. Nurses love it. Doctors take more convincing. The mention of palliative care can make doctors cringe, especially surgeons. I think that when we mention palliative care, they think we're just giving up. Many physicians feel that they went into medicine to fix problems and to get people better. And admitting that we've gone as far as we can in one or multiple areas and we need to refocus and change our goals can feel like failure to them. However, we always need to advocate whatever is best for the patient.

One of the great things about a palliative care team is they get everyone on the same page. They talk to physicians (which is very helpful when there are multiple doctors involved) and also talk to the family as a whole and assist with decision-making. They are great for painting a complete and consistent picture of prognosis, after given direction from the primary physicians.

Also, when a physician decides to consult palliative care or hospice, make sure that physician tells the family what they're doing. If without warning a palliative care doctor or hospice nurse practitioner comes in and talks to them, that can really set someone off. I've been there. I've seen it happen. I had to try to smooth it over, but ultimately that physician lost all trust, credibility, and respect from a family going through something terrible. Make sure the doctor talks to the family about this, no matter how uncomfortable it may be for them.

Keep in mind, certain religions do not believe at all in hospice or palliative care. I've had a few devout Muslim patients who believe in the longevity of life. They fought for every single day that their loved one had on this earth, even if he or she was in pain and suffering. Granted, that is not the majority of patients, but I had to keep their beliefs ahead of my own personal opinions. While the option of palliative and hospice care should still be presented, be aware they may not respond positively. And that's okay; our opinions don't really matter if that's what the patient would want.

Your tone should change a little bit after the goals of care have shifted from recovery to comfort. I don't know how to describe it, but just be more comforting, supportive, and reassuring rather than motivating and gung-ho with high spirits. These patients (if they're awake) and families are very emotional, understandably so. Don't act differently if they cry. It's okay to hug them. That took me a while to be comfortable with. But once I watched a nurse I really looked up to go and hug a crying wife, I felt reassured that it was okay. And that wife hugged her and cried so hard, but man, she really needed to. And she was so thankful that nurse hugged her first. She was now her go-to person for everything.

A lot of times we're at a loss for words when dealing with these patients and families. We just don't know how to talk to them all of a sudden. That's okay; it's not a comfortable place to be. But we still need to be there for them. Sitting in silence with them is okay.

Something that I have learned that goes a long way is just acknowledging what's going on.

"Mr. Smith, I just want you to know that I'm really sorry that you're going through this."

That says, "I'm here with you, I acknowledge this sucks, but we're going to walk through this and I'll be here to support you today." It can be a small amount of reassurance during a really rough time.

A lot of times, families will think that taking the comfort care step means we have lost all hope. But what hope looks like changes when you walk through life and death. When they were admitted, the hope was that they'd go home. When they had the huge stroke, the hope was that they wouldn't need a feeding tube. When they became unresponsive, the hope was that they would regain consciousness. And when nothing can be done to get the patient home, functioning, and off of a ventilator and multiple vasoactive drips, the hope now becomes being comfortable. Hope doesn't go away. It just changes.

You're not going to make them feel better or take the pain away, you just need to be comforting and supporting. I also have told families that, although this is a terrible situation, I have seen patients pass with no one at their side, and that I think it's wonderful that so many people clearly loved this person.

More than anything, these families want you to empathize with them. They do not want sympathy from you. They don't want you looking down at them while towering over them, patting them on the back telling them everything will be okay. They want you to sit next to them and connect with them. Nothing you say will fix what's happening. Let go of that desire (much easier said than done). Be content and comfortable sitting next to them while they're crying, and connect with them. "I'm so sorry you're going through this," goes a long, long way.

Once you do it a few times, you'll get better, but it never gets easy. You may also get a lot of, "Why would God allow this?" and "Why is God taking them away from me?" kinds of questions. Everyone's comfort level with that is different. A standard, "I don't know; I'm so sorry" is always okay because, really, how can you ever begin to answer that?

Being a Christian, I have prayed with patients and their families before. Keep in mind; this was only after I had the green green green light after multiple unprovoked conversations about their beliefs and God's role in their life. So if you feel comfortable, and they have given you the green light without you mentioning anything at all first, go for it. I'll never forget those patients; they were so thankful for that support and will always, always have a place in my heart. Some of the sweetest cards came from them. They made me cry weeks later!

If you're not comfortable with all that God stuff, which is more than fine, call the chaplain to support them spiritually. They are awesome. And if the family doesn't connect with that particular denomination or person, they'll know whom to contact to get the right one there.

Also, when you're around someone who is actively grieving, please remember that silence is okay. Don't feel like you need to say the perfect reassuring thing to them. Nothing you say is going to fix what's happening. Your job in that moment is to support them, not make them feel better with the perfect thing to say. Sit with them, comfort them, and empathize with them. I used to feel like I had to come up with the perfect thing to say when someone was crying in front of me, but now I realize that it's not what I say that will comfort them, it's more about my presence and support. This speaks much louder than any words.

Being there for those patients and families is tough, and even if you feel like you haven't helped at all, that's okay. You probably have and had no idea. They'll probably never forget you. They may not remember your name, but they will probably never forget the nurse who was there for them when their loved one died.

So tell them you're sorry, tell them you're here for them, grab them some tissues, let them cry on your shoulder, hug them, don't be afraid of them, and if they want some prayer from you, go for it. They'll be forever thankful for your support.

And even if you don't know what the heck to say to them, just take really, really good care of their loved one. That will always be enough, because that's all they really want.

CHAPTER 8

The Shift That Broke Me

Have you ever had a shift in which afterwards you didn't know how you'd be able to return to work? I had one of those. It brought me to my knees, it hurt so much. It was a life-changing 12 hours.

I walked into the intensive care unit like any other day. I looked at the assignment sheet and saw I only had one patient. That could only mean one of two things. It meant that either God shined down on me that morning and I only had one patient that day, or it meant that this patient was so time consuming that I would need all of my energy and focus on only that one.

I typically get assigned the patients that are knocking on death's door, or the patients with family members who need a lot of emotional attention. I'm not sure if that's a blessing or a curse, but it's part of the job.

I walked over to see the intubated 50-something gentleman. My eyes narrowed as I stared at his face. I got an eerie feeling.

After a second, I realized why looking at him was so disturbing for me. He looked a little like my husband.

The family had just stepped out during report. It's always weird seeing people with breathing tubes with a normal face and in good shape. They just look so... normal.

Normal-looking people are not so normal in the intensive care world. People are usually swollen or pale or have cuts/abrasions on their face. They look emaciated. Many look poorly kept.

But not this guy. He looked like what I picture my husband will look like in 20 years, but with a breathing tube. It was quite surreal to see.

The night nurse went through her report. He basically had a stroke in the worst part of the brain to get one—the brainstem. You cannot live without your brainstem. It tells your heart to beat, it tells your lungs to breathe. Without it, you will die. And he had a blood clot get into his brain stem and cut off the blood supply.

I looked at him and sighed deeply, thinking about what the next 12 hours would entail.

Apparently that morning he went outside to water his plants in the backyard before work and collapsed. His wife was out of town for work, not due to be back until that afternoon. When he didn't show up for work, his co-workers got worried. A friend drove over and found him. After the stroke hit, he lost all control over his extremities. He was instantly paralyzed. He lay there for 2.5 hours.

He was immediately intubated and brought to my hospital, where they quickly tried to retrieve the clot to prevent more damage. It had been so long since it occurred, the damage had already been done. There was nothing we could do to fix it. Once brain cells die, they die. There's no getting back what has been lost.

That all had happened yesterday, and overnight, he became unstable. Whenever you have a stroke, your brain swells. With him, it wasn't if it was going to swell, it was when. And with a stroke in his brainstem, we were very worried about him *herniating* and then becoming *brain dead*.

> ***Nurse-ipedia definition:*** *Brain death is when you no longer have brain function. It is irreversible and in most states when someone is declared brain dead, they are legally dead. Herniation is when the blood vessels, CSF, and/or brain are pushed from an increase in pressure away from their usual place in the skull. Brain herniation can result in brain death.*

The night nurse was fighting tears giving me report. She felt like there was something she could have done to prevent it, but there wasn't. Fixing this and preventing these inevitable complications that we were beginning to see was beyond what medicine could do.

She told me about his wife that loved him so much it made me feel nauseated. Not nauseated in the, *oh great, you guys are so cute it makes me sick,* way. Nauseated in the, *you're about to lose your best friend for the last 29 years right in front of me and you don't know it yet,* way.

When his wife walked in the room, I could see how exhausted she was. Up for the last 36 hours and enduring the most emotional pain she had ever had to endure was taking its toll. One minute she was finishing up a work conference, the next she was getting a crash course in neurology. Complex medical language was coming her way faster than she could handle.

She walked into the room with a look on her face like she had a knife in her stomach. Sick, nauseated, in pain, dazed, and confused. She wasn't happy to see a new face this early in the morning. She wasn't happy she had to learn another person's name.

With bloodshot eyes, she reluctantly introduced herself to me.

I completed a full neurological assessment and it was about as grim as it could get. He had no basic, primal reflexes. He did not have a cough or gag reflex. He didn't even have a corneal reflex (I could touch his cornea with cotton or saline and he wouldn't even attempt to close his eyes.) His pupils were barely reactive. When I opened his eyes, his eyes *bobbed downward*. They didn't focus on me, or anything; they just bobbed. When I checked to see how his arms and legs responded, I had to elicit pain because he wouldn't move when I asked him to. Even with extreme pain, his arms and legs just laid there, lifeless. He had nothing.

> *Nurse-ipedia explanation: when someone's eyes bob and don't track or focus on anyone, it indicates brain stem involvement of their injury, which is a very ominous sign.*

So there he laid, with a breathing tube in, no sedation, no reflexes, and no hope for recovery. His wife sat next to his bedside, staring at him. Occasionally she'd run her hand through his hair, looking at him longingly. His sons came in and sat next to him on the bed. One leaned over and started talking to him.

The phone rang and it was the neurologist. I told him my assessment. He told me that the patient was probably in a "locked in" like condition. He wouldn't regain function; he wouldn't progress to brain death (he wouldn't swell enough to herniate and cause complete brain death and therefore death). He would just be. He would be dependent on a ventilator forever, if he survived. He would live in a nursing home forever and never be able to do anything except be aware of what's going on around him, but not be able to communicate. He would feel pain and know what's going on around him; he just wouldn't be able to do anything about it. Some people with locked-in syndrome can blink to communicate and breathe on their own. Not him.

"Well, let's get an MRI to see the extent of the damage so I can talk to the family about prognosis and make some decisions today," the neurologist said. I put the order in and let the family know the plan.

"I'll take him downstairs to get an MRI so we can get a really good and detailed picture so the neurologist can go over it with you guys," I said.

She quietly said, "Okay," as she stroked his hand.

I just looked at her as my heart sank into my stomach. I was fighting back tears and it was only 0812. She looked the way I would look if it were my husband in that bed. The look on her face told me how deeply she loved him. The waiting room with over 40 people in it told me how much everyone else loved him. I tried to compartmentalize all of the thoughts going through my head, because if I was overly emotional, I wouldn't be able to take care of either of them.

"He is my best friend," she said through a new batch of tears. "I shouldn't have gone to that conference. I would have been there," she said as she was shaking her head in disappointment.

I didn't know what to say. I didn't know how to respond. I honestly didn't want to. I wanted to run away and go take care of the patient who was getting ready to go to the floor later in the day. I wasn't prepared for this emotional day.

I sat next to her, put my hand on her back and all I could think to say was, "I'm sorry. I am so, so sorry."

After a few minutes, I got up and left her alone with him. I went to quickly chart my assessment, grab the meds that were due and the monitor I had to take him downstairs on, and came back. There she was, still staring at him.

While I got things together, people came in and out, all with that same face. The kind of face where you can tell they're using all that's in them not to cry. Their two sons were the worst for me to see, after his wife. One was older (I think mid-20's, not sure) and less emotional. He was trying to be strong for his mom and brother. The younger son was past trying to look strong. His heart had been ripped out and he didn't know what to do with it.

I packed him up and started wheeling him out of the room and off the unit. The patient's long-time friend stopped me. "Can I come down with him? I don't want him to be alone."

"Of course you can," I said. "There's an MRI waiting room I'll have you wait in while he's in the scanner."

"Ok, that'll be fine. I just really don't want him to be alone," he said with a quiver in his voice.

He almost got me. Even when I try to have my strongest Nurse Face on, men who cry just penetrate my defenses and get to me. Miraculously, I held it together.

It was a quiet elevator ride and quiet trip to the MRI suite. I put his friend in the waiting room and brought him into the room and greeted the MRI techs.

To get an MRI of the brain, you have to lay flat in the scanner. Now when you lay down flat, the pressure slightly increases in your brain because of gravity. Not a problem for us, but it's a problem for a guy with an acute stroke in his brainstem in which we're worried about swelling.

I laid him flat, and initially he was okay. I had an MRI compatible monitor on him so I could closely monitor his vitals while he was in the scanner.

As I sat there, outside the scanning room, looking in at his monitor through the large window, I saw his heart rate begin to drop. All of a sudden, his heart was 38, his blood pressure was 190s, and he was covered in sweat.

"I NEED TO SIT HIM UP! He's starting to herniate!" I yelled to the MRI techs as they ran to let me into the room. I sat him up and yelled for someone to grab *atropine*. If his heart rate didn't come back up after I relieved the pressure on his brain, we were going to have a brain dead man on our hands in a matter of moments. Apparently, his brain couldn't handle the small amount of added pressure of laying flat for more than a few minutes. Not a good sign.

> *Nurse-ipedia definition: atropine is an ACLS medication used to increase the heart rate when it drops very low and the patient has symptoms (or symptomatic bradycardia) that can include dizziness, sweating, fainting, and chest pains.*

Thankfully, his heart rate quickly came back up and his vitals stabilized with the change in position.

The MRI tech helped me rush him back up to the unit, grabbing his friend on the way.

I didn't want to explain it all to his friend before I explained it to his wife. As we were walking, I was putting the words together in my mind to tell her what happened, and why the scan I told her would take an hour only took nine minutes.

"His brain couldn't handle the pressure of lying flat. We won't be able to get a scan on him."

Through tears he asked, "What does that mean?"

"I don't know," I lied. "I have to talk to the neurologist."

As I started getting closer to the unit, his wife saw me, and suddenly her face looked puzzled as she quickly started walking towards us.

"Let me get him settled and hooked back up, and I'll meet you back here to tell you what's going on," I said as she nodded her head. "Someone page neurology STAT for me," I said as I wheeled him back to his room.

Another nurse saw me coming back into the unit way earlier than expected and came to see what happened as she helped me get him back on our monitors.

"His heart rate dropped, pressure skyrocketed, and he got diaphoretic," I told her.

"Oh God," she said. She'd worked in this unit for almost a decade. She knew what that meant. I didn't need to tell her anything else. I did another neuro assessment, which was unchanged from the previous one. She told me something ridiculous that another patient did, which calmed my nerves and made me forget the fact that I was buttoning up the gown of an almost brain dead man who looked just like my husband. Thank the Lord for my nursey coworkers.

The phone rang. It was the neurologist answering my page. I told him what happened in MRI.

"Given the location of the stroke and his assessment, I expected him to be unstable down there. I guess we can't do a scan. I'll be there in about an hour; I'm finishing with a few other patients."

All I could mutter was, "Okay."

I was tired, frustrated, and confused. The emotional ups and downs of the day were starting to get to me. I was frustrated that I wasn't warned by the physician, who had already known what would most likely happen, and confused as to why it was ordered in the first place. At this point in the day, getting upset about this wasn't going to provide any relief; it would just make me more frustrated. I took a few deep breaths and put it behind me.

I walked out to his wife just outside of the unit in the hallway who was anxiously awaiting my return.

"What happened!?" she asked.

I explained to her that I laid him flat, and he became unstable because of the pressure in his brain. His heart rate dropped really low, he got sweaty, and I had to immediately set him up to relieve the pressure; and because of that we couldn't get the scan.

"If we just give him some time, can we just try again later?" she asked with the last ounce of hope in her eyes.

I paused for a second. I should have told her we needed to wait for the doctor to know. All of the "I should haves" still run through my mind to this day. I was tired of pretending I didn't know things. Tired of seeing that little bit of hope in her eyes.

"No," I said. "And it'll just continue to get worse."

That was it. That's when it hit her that he was gone.

She immediately clung to me and started sobbing into my scrubs. She held on to me so tight, I lost my breath for a moment. Some family and friends ran up to her once they saw her so upset. She was so distraught she almost passed out. Not quite, but oh so close. I grabbed a chair as she stumbled to it with the help of a few loved ones. With her family comforting her and her now safely sitting in a chair, I took a beeline out of there. I was now in survival mode. "If I start sobbing right now, I cannot continue," I thought. I could hear her sobbing loudly as I raced to the restroom, tears filling my eyes and pouring down my cheeks.

The other nurses knew. They knew what was going on. They knew she just got hit in the face with a death punch. They knew how hard it was for me because they had all seen it themselves. And they, understandably so, were just thankful it wasn't them today.

As I got closer to the bathroom, one of the nurses gave me a reassuring pat on the back. I was thankful for his gesture, even though it made me more emotional.

I closed the door and sat on the nasty bathroom floor and sobbed. I couldn't hold myself up anymore. I was done. I turned on the water and cried louder. It took about five minutes for me to cry and compose myself. My makeup was gone; I looked like hell, but whatever. That was the last thing on my mind. I blew my nose one more time, took a few deep breaths, and walked out of the bathroom.

I went back to his room to do another assessment, and to turn him, when I saw the neurologist walk onto the floor. I went to go talk with him privately before he spoke with the family.

When I saw him, we gave each other the, "This really, really sucks" look. I talked to him, forgetting the whole sending me down for an MRI thing, and he basically said that their options were to let him be locked-in, or let him pass. Normally, I would sit in on this conversation; however, I was at my emotional breaking point and couldn't take it anymore. I had a feeling I knew what their decision would be, and therefore knew how the rest of the day was going to play out. I was in survival mode.

I sat this one out.

He took her and a few close family members into the family conference room to deliver the final blow. It took about 20 minutes. I used that time to bathe him, assess him (which was again unchanged), and just be away from it for a bit to collect myself.

Sometimes these situations come to you with a decision already made. They're already so far gone that there isn't a choice for the family. However, there was a choice this time, and it was cut and dry. There were two options, and both were rip-your-heart-out terrible.

When you look at him, he's breathing (only because there's a ventilator breathing for him). His heart is beating. He has a blood pressure. He looks very alive. You look at him and think, "Let's just give him some time to come around and see what happens... let's give him a chance." And sometimes, that's perfectly appropriate; however, not with this guy. He was going to either be in a nursing home forever, feeling pain, getting bedsores and pneumonia. He would be aware of it, but not able to do anything about it; not able to communicate, not able to control his bladder or bowels, and having a permanent feeding and breathing tube, or, he could meet his Maker.

Those conversations are tough for everyone, including the physicians. Delivering that kind of news, you feel like an angel of death. And sometimes they don't understand when the doctor tells them, so you as the nurse, have to gracefully reinforce what the doctor said. Your job is to be realistic; you don't want to lie to them and give them false hope. It's your job to be honest with them.

I walked back to his room, and when I turned the corner into the room, I felt my heart sink to my stomach. There she was, lying in the bed with him, sobbing on his chest.

That ripped my heart out. If I were her, I would have done the same thing. If someone just told me my husband was gone, I'd be right there, lying next to him, sobbing on his chest.

I gave her some time. I came back after a little while and sat and talked with her. She told me stories about him being her best friend, and the best father and provider she could have ever hoped and prayed for. Multiple people came in and out, crying. This man had a profound and positive effect on so many people.

They spoke with the neurologist again and decided to let him pass. It was hard to say how long he would last off of the breathing tube, so we decided to transfer him to the hospice unit.

Typically, we transport the patient from our unit to the hospice unit and remove the breathing tube once we arrive. We do this because we don't want someone to *fly* and stay in the busy and loud intensive care unit for days while slowly dying when we thought it was going to be a quick process. Additionally, we don't want to remove the breathing tube before we transfer them and have them pass away en route to the next room.

Nurse ipedia definition: When a breathing tube is removed and someone does well off of the ventilator, we say that they fly... like a little bird with tiny wings that you didn't expect to get in the air.

I always dread those cases because taking them down there and leaving them, knowing they'll die, is just really hard.

We secured a bed, and I gave report. Myself, the respiratory therapist, and his wife walked in silence as we bagged him down to the hospice unit.

Once we got there, we wheeled him into the room. When the wife, kids, mom, and siblings were in the room and ready, we took his tube out. He was breathing. Technically.

I gave his wife and kids hugs and tried not to sob.

As I looked over to get one last glance of him, I saw him take his last breath.

He suddenly no longer looked like that perfectly normal guy with a breathing tube. He looked like what little life was left in him had gone. Peacefully.

The color immediately drained from his face. I quickly exited the room for that intimate moment. I let out a few tears as I raced past the 30 people in the hallway. I could hear the loud sobs of the people at the bedside all the way down by the nurse's station. I let the hospice nurse know that he passed and needed to be pronounced. I left as quickly as I possibly could.

My day started with getting report on him at 0700 and ended with his death at 1800.

When I got back up to the unit, it was about 20 minutes from shift change. There was already another patient on the way to take his spot. Thankfully, they would arrive after shift change and I wouldn't have to take report. I don't know if I could have at that point. I was trying really hard not to cry those last 20 minutes.

Whenever something like that happens, all the other nurses just know. They know the mood shifts. They know you're on the verge of tears. They know your heart just got ripped out. It's so good to be part of that team because we've all been there. We've all had those patients. And whenever you have one, or they know you just got done doing something really, really tough… there's this reassuring look they all give you. It's one of those, "You're a good nurse, hang in there, we're in this together," looks.

The nurse who took care of him the night before was back. I told her what happened and she wanted to go down to hospice with me to go see him and the family really quickly. I knew it'd be rough, but I felt that it would be good to go see the family one last time.

We went down there and saw everyone. The wife was at his side with a look of peace. She was very calm. His mother sobbed as she hugged me and called me an angel. His brother, a huge farmer, said thank you through his tears. My coworker and I just were trying to hold it together. We let a few tears sneak out, just enough to keep us from losing it altogether.

We walked back and replayed the last 24 hours in the elevator. We reassured each other. We supported each other. That situation bonded us greatly. We walked through the depths of a family's worst nightmare together.

I went home that night and sobbed on my husband's chest. This now felt like a luxury, not an expectation.

I finally cried the tears that I'd been holding in all day.

For a few weeks, I dreamt about them. I saw his face in my dreams with that breathing tube and his bobbing eyes. I saw his wife sobbing on his chest. I felt her cling to me when she found out he was gone. I saw his last breath. I heard his family sob down the hallway.

Those situations are hard to process, and it was my first experience with something like that. Thankfully, my next couple shifts were easy, straight forward and happy.

Sometimes when someone passes we try to go to the funeral. I couldn't handle being there, so myself, and a few others, sent some flowers.

A week later, my husband and I went to our weekly Bible study. In our women's small group, I shared the situation. I started sobbing all over again. One by one, everyone prayed for me. As they did, I felt a release. I felt a peace that I hadn't felt since.

I didn't dream about him anymore after that. It was like God had a purpose for me in that situation and with that family, and wanted to release me of the pain that came along with it.

Looking back, I'm thankful I had the privilege of caring for him and his family that day, even though it was one of the hardest things I've ever done. I know there was purpose in me being there, and am thankful that I could be. I am humbled to be the one that got to be there for them.

I thought that shift was going to break me. And it did. It broke me in a grace-filled way. It broke me in a, *I'm so thankful for all that I have,* way.

It broke me in a way that made me more compassionate and empathetic, and present both physically and emotionally for my family, friends, and patients. Being broken for your patients allows you to enter into what they're experiencing. It enables you to really be present for them, and therefore really care for them in the way they need it most.

CHAPTER 9

If It Makes You Feel Any Better

Man, that was rough – wasn't it!? This chapter is more light-hearted. I promise.

When going through nursing school, meeting new coworkers, and living the full-blown nursey life, everyone wants to be the best possible nurse they can be. They want to project that image to everyone so that everyone thinks they're competent and never mess up.

If you ask any seasoned nurse about the biggest mistake they've made, it usually starts a hilarious and interesting conversation. These nurses are typically secure in themselves, and can admit the mistakes that have made them better. And it makes you feel more human as a newbie that there are not these unrealistic expectations.

(Note: nurses that say they haven't made mistakes are liars.)

In addition to making mistakes, ridiculous things happen to us. Some so ridiculous, they're difficult to believe. I also think it's important to be reminded that we're human. Just because we've gone through nursing school doesn't mean we don't get scared, anxious, angry, or upset. We're expected to deal with things as they arise with professionalism and grace, however on the inside we may be terrified or freaking out. And that's okay. We've all been there.

I wrote this next section to let you know that you're not alone. It's okay to have emotions. It's okay to be scared, tired, frustrated angry, or embarrassed. I've been there. I've walked through it, and it does get better.

So, if it makes you feel any better...

I had those mini panic attacks before work.

I freaked out every time I had to call a doctor.

I cried in the bathroom the first time a doctor yelled at me.

I cried after a terrible day in the car on the way home.

I called a patient's wife his mother.

I took report on the wrong patient.

I had to admit a med error to an attending physician and four of her residents. (It was minor with no ill-effects, but still embarrassing nonetheless.)

I stood at the door and watched a patient and his mother scream at each other because I was too terrified to do anything about it.

A patient call 911 on me. She was admitted for cholecysitis and confusion, so whenever she would eat anything she would be in terrible pain but forget that the food caused the pain. We did not allow her food or drink on admission and started IV fluids. She later called 911 from her hospital bed and told them we were starving her and didn't remember the many conversations we had.

I had to implement and order for "scrotal elevation" on a man with a "scrotum the size of a soccer ball."

I've had to digitally disimpact way more patients than I'd like to admit.

I asked a patient with bilateral above the knee amputations where her socks were. (I swear I had no idea. She had a blanket on…)

I spent an hour doing a complex dressing change just to have the physician come by and rip it off and not tell me.

I've had to dig feces out from under a patient's nails.

I stayed late because I hadn't charted a word until 1930…and I ended up leaving at 2100.

I was terrified when I floated the first time, but it wasn't so bad.

I froze during my first code.

I had to change my scrubs after my confused patient pooped so much that he created a "poop slide" and slid down and out of the bed and hit the floor. Actually, three of us had to change our scrubs.

I called my mom after every shift to tell her all the gross and cool things I'd done from my first nursing clinical to … yesterday. (Being HIPAA compliant, of course!)

I survived a shift off of saltines, peanut butter, and ginger ale because I didn't have time to stop.

I've lost it at the nurse's station multiple times when a patient who was on death's door walked back onto the unit a month later just to to tell us 'thank you'.

I wasted a lot of time doing patient care and getting behind on my charting, because I was too scared to delegate to the tech playing on her phone.

I had to get respectfully assertive with a patient who called me stupid and put her finger in my face.

I brought a patient in to see his father with dementia, and after an hour his sister walked by the room and saw him talking to the wrong man. The son insisted it was his father until his sister walked him to the room next to him and showed him his actual father. And this was after the patient's "son" convinced him to let us do a test we had been trying to get done all morning.

I sprayed tube-feeding residual all over myself, and my patient, because I forgot to flip the stopcock.

I felt anxious every day before work, but with each shift it got better.

I accidentally pulled out a patient's external pacing wire before it was indicated when he was standing up from the recliner.

I'm still not the best IV starter in the unit years later, but there's more to nursing than that.

I still ask questions every single day.

Being in charge of someone's care for 12 hours at a time can be scary. But as you walk through various experiences, you become more confident. I think it's important to know that you're not alone in this journey. Even if people pretend like they're fine after something scary happens or they're not mad or sad when someone was just really demeaning to them, it still affects us. Being aware of that within each other can help us to better support one another as we're growing into awesome nurses. So ask for help or support when you are in need and be there for others when they're going through something as well. We're all on the same team!

Every nurse has these stories. We all screw up and figure out how to do things better the next time. Your first few years are full of these moments that eventually turn into hilarious, heartbreaking, empowering, or frustrating stories. One of my more hilarious stories from my beginnings that I look back to with laughter and frustration was when I got poop on my face.

Yes, you read that right.

The New Nurse, the New CNA, the Traumatic Brain Injury Patient, and the Poop that Touched My Face

After a certain amount of time on your unit, you won't be the most inexperienced person anymore. New people will start to work, and suddenly they will be coming to you for advice. It's quite an eerie feeling.

It was one of those first few shifts where people were coming to me for advice. At this point, I still felt everyone knew more than me. One of my patients was a younger guy (around 40) who was in a car accident a few weeks ago. He was sitting at a stoplight and someone hit him. Among multiple fractures, he had a traumatic brain injury. This made him completely not himself. He could no longer care for himself. He needed to be turned, bathed, and fed. It was truly heart breaking to see him like that while his wife looked at him helplessly.

At this point, he had been in the hospital for approximately two weeks. He had to have multiple surgeries to repair his various fractures, and they were waiting on an inpatient rehab bed. Due to multiple rounds of general anesthesia and intermittent pain medication, this man had not had a bowel movement since before his accident two weeks prior.

His wife came to the nurse's station to let me know that she thought he had gone to the bathroom. I gathered supplies and asked a CNA to help me. I'd seen this CNA a few times before, and, being new myself, I just assumed she had much more experience with cleaning and changing people. Oh, how wrong I was.

The man was on contact isolation so every time we went into his room, we had to wear a gown and gloves. Prior to going in, I gathered all supplies, gowned up, and double-gloved.

Typically when we do poopy bed changes, I ask the family to step out. I do this just because it gets pretty gross and most people can't handle it. I really don't want to have to deal with being dirty and have a family member pass out or throw up. I've got enough patients; I don't need another one!

However, this patient's wife insisted on staying in the room. When people insist, I don't push back. I completely understand not wanting to leave your husband's side.

We had everything we needed and got started. With each of us on one side of his bed, we held him up on his side, toward my CNA.

Now, keep in mind that this man had not defecated in about two weeks. We had officially opened the floodgates and there was a countywide flash flood alert. There was such an exorbitant amount of stool that it pooled in the bed under him.

So, we were in our contact isolation gowns that cause any person, whether they are holding up a 200lb man or not, to immediately start sweating. Honestly, I probably should start working out in those things because minimal movements produce significant perspiration.

After about five minutes of inefficiently cleaning (give me a break, I was still new!), beads of sweat were pouring down my face. I had already gone through both gloves and double-gloved again. Unable to bear more sweat getting into my eyes and clouding my contacts, I inspected my gloves and gowned sleeve. My gloves were new and my gown hadn't touched the patient at all. I thought I was good. I thought I was safe. I couldn't bear it any longer, so I wiped my forehead with my sleeve.

I immediately felt something across my face that did not feel like the gown.

"Oh my God! Is it on my face?! Did I get it on my face!?" I frantically asked the tech standing across from me, forgetting the patient's wife was in the room.

"No, no you're good," she said as she closely inspected my face.

Feeling relieved, I continued cleaning.

After struggling through the rest of the bed change, I ran to the bathroom to look in the mirror. I know she said I was okay, but I just didn't believe her.

And there it was. A poop stripe was on my right cheek, just inches from my eye, like eye black on a football player's face.

I immediately grabbed soap and water and scrubbed it off my face. I topped it off with a few deep scrubs from a handful of alcohol swabs to insure optimal cleanliness.

Too embarrassed to admit it to my coworkers at the nurse's station, I just told them about how much poop there was... not that any physically came into contact with my face. As I was talking, one of them pointed at my shoulder and said in a disgusted voice, "What is that? Is that stool?"

I looked down and there it was...another stripe of stool on my shoulder.

Never getting bodily fluids on my scrubs before, I didn't know what to do. Like a frantic child, I looked to the more experienced nurses for my next step. "What do I do!? I don't have another scrub top here!"

"Call the OR," they all said in unison, with grossed-out looks on all of their faces. (When a group of nurses is grossed-out, you KNOW it's bad.) Most hospitals have a plethora of scrubs that you can wear, should yours become compromised. Typically, it's the operating room/surgical services department because they have to wear in-house scrubs in their department. They're always ill fitting, and you look like a big blue blob. They're not ideal but they're better than poop scrubs.

And so for the first time, I called down to the OR to get a replacement set of scrubs. For those of you who aren't nurses, the first time that you have to get a new set of scrubs because someone crapped, peed, puked, or bled on you is one of those nursing-initiation things. Kind of like the first time you resuscitate someone after a code, or the first time you get an awesome IV on a confused patient, or the first time you do CPR.

Again, welcome to the wonderful world of nursing

CHAPTER 10

Life After Work

Nursing is an all-encompassing career. We may not physically take work home with us after a shift, but we take our patients home with us in our hearts. We hear IV pumps, telemetry alarms, bed alarms, feeding pumps, and phones ringing in our sleep. We see the faces of the patients we coded in our dreams. We hear the sobs and screams of distraught family members when we're trying to relax after a terrible day.

Nursing is very selfless. Our patients are always before us. We see something terribly sad in one room, and then something incredibly exciting and happy in the next, and we have to behave accordingly. We stuff down tears when we're trying to be professional during a tough conversation. We hide laughter when a patient refuses to wear a gown and insists on being naked. We swallow our extreme frustration when a patient throws out unreasonable demand after unreasonable demand, treating us as their servants. We sit back when a patient's family ignores us and sings the physician's praises after their loved one has punched, bit, kicked, and cursed at us for the last eight hours.

This career is so hard because we care. It's not just about meeting a financial goal or outperforming last year. It's about the patients and their families. It's about caring for people going through something terrible. It's just about being there for people. You don't get into a career where cleaning poop is part of the job description if you don't care.

Even if we had all of the time in the world to care for our patients, with the best equipment and the most supportive management and medical teams, it would still be hard. People would still die and we would still be there, holding their hands. Doing that tough emotional stuff isn't easy, but we do it because someone else needs it.

The Importance of Your Nursey Voice

Nursing is, always has been, and always will be, a forever-changing field. Because change happens quickly and frequently, we have to be in constant communication with those around us. Some changes are fantastic and really streamline bedside care. Sometimes things that sound like a good idea actually aren't when you get to the bedside.

If it is something that I feel very strongly about, I talk about it with my assistant manager, my manager, or my unit Shared Governance council. There's no need to talk negatively about the change or leadership/management, and not bring it to the source or to a platform that can influence change. Gossiping about something you don't like is counterproductive and makes for a terrible work environment, and before you know it, you'll be the cancer of the entire unit. You'll turn into the person that people see on the schedule and feel they have to mentally prepare themselves to work with because of the negativity.

Something that's important to me is being able to have a say in the decisions that affect how I provide patient care. I also want to be up to date on all of the procedures and polices that are ever-evolving. To do this, I've become involved in Shared Governance at both places I've worked. These councils are where change occurs. They are where information is disseminated. They are where you have a voice. If there is a process that needs improving, bring it there. Please do not talk about how terrible a process is if you're not willing to try to change it. You are at the front lines and people in leadership need your opinion. Those councils are where your nursey voice is heard. I beg you to speak.

However, keep in mind that not all of your ideas or suggestions will be acted upon. While we're at the bedside, the leadership has to have the big picture in mind, which almost always consists of aspects of problems that we, as bedside nurses, do not consider. We must express our concerns and suggestions as appropriate but also realize that not everything is doable.

Something I highly respect about the experienced nurses on our floor is that regardless of how they feel about whatever change is occurring, they all hold each other accountable. If someone is taking a shortcut or doing what he or she shouldn't be, you'll hear someone say, "You know I love you, but that's not right and you know it." And before you know it, they've changed their negative behavior and everything is fine. No one treats each other poorly after that, no one's relationship changes. I think that's why our team works so well together. We hold each other to high standards and always put the patient first. And there are no favorites; everyone is held to the same standard regardless of how many years people have been there. I really love and respect my coworkers.

The Work-Life Balance

Striking a healthy work-life balance in the nursing profession is quite challenging, but absolutely essential. It takes a lot of trial and error to figure out what works for each individual person. You'll know you've found it when you discover a balance that is sustainable. You feel not only professional, but personal satisfaction in what you do to earn your living.

When I wake up the morning of work, I leave enough time for myself and my husband to read a devotional and our Bibles together, and pray before we start our day. This allows us to start our day together on a positive note. If we are not on the top of our game, or need specific prayer, we make sure to cover each other in it before stepping out of the door. Keeping my heart and head focused on God keeps all that I do, at work and at home, in perspective.

I also pray on my way to work to get my mind right. I pray for peace, strength, discernment, and just to be a good nurse and coworker. Truly, I believe that the reason I can walk into this stressful and emotional job with peace and joy every single day is because He gives that so graciously to me. I thank Jesus for His sacrifice. I thank Him that I have a job and my health, and I thank Him for my loved ones' health. Working with stroke patients who suddenly lose basic functions constantly keeps this on the forefront of my mind. Walking in every day humbled and thankful keeps my heart and mind ready for whatever may come my way. It just keeps me at peace.

With each and every day I work, I try to do the best I can with what I've been given while I'm there. That allows me mentally to "leave it all on the court," as the saying goes. I do the best I can, and if I've done that, there's no use worrying or stressing about what more I could have done. I take care of my patients and their loved ones like they are my family, and really, that's all anyone can ask you to do.

If I screw up, I let my one-up know, and write myself up if I need to. I learn what I need to learn and move on.

I help my coworkers, I manage my time, and I communicate with every-one throughout the day. I maintain respect for every single person I work with, and expect the same from them. If something changes at work that dissatisfies the staff, I try to take it in stride. Change is inevitable and will continue to happen in this field. Getting upset about each and every change creates unnecessary worry and stress.

My husband and I try to get away and take a weekend trip together a few times a year. Every year, we pick a game (like a card or board game) and play it a few times a week and keep a count of wins. Whoever loses has to plan a weekend getaway. My husband lost, of course, this last year and took me to Charleston, SC. We went to a restaurant featured on the Food Network and I ate the most delicious fried chicken I had ever tasted. It put all other fried chicken to shame. There, I definitely wasn't thinking about a rude patient with an unreasonable family member. And we turned off our cell phones when we got there. It was glorious.

And if we can't go on a real weekend trip away, we will have a stay-cation and just cut ourselves off from work, but relax at home together. I think if you make this a priority, it not only reduces your stress, but also enhances your relationship.

We try to make time at least every other week to spend with friends and family. We host game nights, go out for karaoke, go wine tasting, or go hiking. I think it's important to cultivate and maintain relationships with people continually throughout your life. If you only see your spouse, your children, and your close family, you can lose touch with the rest of the world and become complacent. It's good to have people surrounding you who will challenge you, hold you accountable, call you out, and get you out of your comfort zone. Life is too short to live in the comfort zone.

I'm not saying your spouse, children, and family cannot do this; there is just something different and valuable about cultivating and maintaining relationships outside of the family dynamic. They can offer support and a point of view that is very different from your family. And honestly, sometimes we need to be supported by people outside of our family so that we ourselves can support our family.

Additionally, something important to be disciplined about when you start nursing are your finances. This is especially important if you've just graduated and have loans. If it's your first job out of college, you'll be getting used to basic financial planning. I highly recommend creating a budget, sticking to it, and living below your means. Financial stress can be quite the burden, and if you start out right and are not strapped for cash immediately, you won't feel the need to constantly pick up overtime. I know this isn't realistic for everyone, but any discipline you can have in this area will pay off.

While nursing provides a great salary, it's not a six-figure salary that will give you that HGTV-ready home, a BMW, and a Pinterest-perfect wardrobe. Figuring my finances took a few years because I had the mentality, "I'm making a lot more now and therefore can afford a lot more". That's not true when you factor in insurances (make sure you get short-term disability insurance!), car payment, mortgage payments, gas, cable/internet, groceries, medical expenses, Netflix (now a non-negotiable budgetary item), and so on. Establish a budget that's below your means, and stick to it!

Establishing a work-life balance is different for everyone, but it is essential for your sanity. If you're working too much, it's not sustainable and you'll be unhappy. If you never work, you'll lose your passion. But honestly, not too many people can afford to never work! I know nursing school was terribly demanding, and learning how to be a nurse is an entirely different kind of stress, but you will find yourself as a nurse.

Thank You

So if you're in nursing school, a practicing nurse, or a retired nurse, thanks. Thank you for what you do or have done. Not everyone has nursing within him or her. Not everyone can handle this.

This career truly requires all of you, and taps into parts of your heart and life that most are not okay with sharing. Thank you for going there. Thank you for *being* there; holding someone's hand as they pass away because their family couldn't get there in time. Thank you for spending time with the teenager dying from cancer. Thank you for helping bring new life into this world. Thank you for delivering that baby because the doctor didn't get there in time. Thank you for allowing people to die with dignity. Just, thank you.

I am honored to be a nurse along with you. It brings me great joy to be able to help you grow as a nurse. I pray this book helped you. And I pray this book will help you help others. I pray that you are more confident not only in your nursing skills, but also in yourself. You are a precious commodity, oh nursey friend of mine. Please take care of yourself.

Stay nursey.

Stay strong.